Safely Home

Also by Julie Shaw Cole

Getting Life, a novel

SAFELY HOME

A Profile of a Futures Planning Group

Compiled by Betty Atherton and Julie Shaw Cole
Edited by Julie Shaw Cole

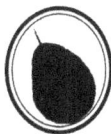

The Advocado Press

Louisville, KY

Safely Home: A Profile of a Futures Planning Group

Published by The Advocado Press, Inc., P.O. Box 145, Louisville, KY 40201
www.advocadopress.org

Library of Congress Cataloging-in-Publication Data

Safely home : a profile of a futures planning group / compiled by Betty Atherton and Julie Shaw Cole ; edited by Julie Shaw Cole.
    p. cm.
 Includes bibliographical references.
 ISBN-13: 978-0-9721189-2-7 (pbk.)
 ISBN-10: 0-9721189-2-6 (pbk.)
1. People with mental disabilities--Institutional care--United States. 2. People with mental disabilities--Services for--United States. 3. Atherton, Raymond, 1966-2002. 4. People with mental disabilities--United States--Biography. 5. People with mental disabilities--Family relationships--United States. 6. Social integration--United States. I. Atherton, Betty. II. Cole, Julie Shaw.
 HV3006.A4S34 2008
 362.3092--dc22
 [B]
                            2008028153

Table of Contents

Chapter 1   **Fish Fry**   **1**

The reason for Raymond's group 2
Raymond's history and childhood medical issues 4
Family life and school experiences 5
What to do next? 9
Circle origins – R.E.A.C.H. and the dream 11
Back to the fish fry 14

Chapter 2   **The Methods of the Circle**   **16**

Futures planning. 16
Graphic facilitation 21
Being committed 24

Chapter 3   **Out REACH**   **27**

Chapter 4   **Reach Out**   **30**

Chapter 5   **Choices?**   **34**

A conversation in the group about choices 36

Chapter 6   **Family Matters**   **42**

Family connection 44

Chapter 7   **Family Supports**   **47**

Family supports beyond family 48

Chapter 8   **Key Chains**   **51**

More invitations to outside support 51
Art therapy 52

Chapter 9   **Antennae – Raymond being himself**   **62**

Chapter 10   **ReModeling – Finding a Place**   **70**

Application to HUD 71
Family involvement 72

Chapter 11   Recruitment   75

Matching people with Raymond 76
Matching Raymond with people 78

Chapter 12   Finding Funding   84

The fine line between institution and community integration 85
Coordinating funding sources 86

An Unpleasant Intermezzo   96

Chapter 13   Working – Making a day for Raymond   101

First case in point. 102
Second case in point: Trial and error. 103
Third case in point: Trial and success 104
Fourth case in point: Success and burnout, Raymond and Jim. 105
Fifth case in point: More trials and more successes 110

Chapter 14   The System?   118

Some thoughts on what the system offers. 118
Work?. 120
Residential services 122
In Raymond's case, there was rarely any talk of "programs" 126

Chapter 15   Safely Home   130

Meeting 1/15/02. 130

Afterword and Dedication, Acknowledgments   136

Appendices   137

Appendix A   Books suggested by members of Raymond's group 138
Appendix B   Glossary. 140
Appendix C   Summary of minutes of Raymond's group. 155
Appendix D   Milton Tyree's notes. 177
Appendix E   Edited notes from art therapy sessions 195
Appendix F   Poems. 207

Chapter 1

Fish Fry

The humidity is so high you can scoop the air up with your hands and pour it on your head. It is August in Kentucky, and the steamy summer evening is tempered by the shade of old-growth oak trees along the road and in the front yard of the trim duplex home. There's a faint breeze, encouraged by the waiting guests fanning paper plates while conversing at long tables set out under the trees. People apply cold soda in sweaty cans and longneck beers from ice-crammed coolers to their heads and mouths to cool down.

In the side yard by the little walkway a canopy shades Gerald, a tall, burly, good-looking guy with bright eyes and a brilliant smile, frying fish in a big flat fryer. He is cheerily sporting a neck and shoulder brace due to a bad accident.

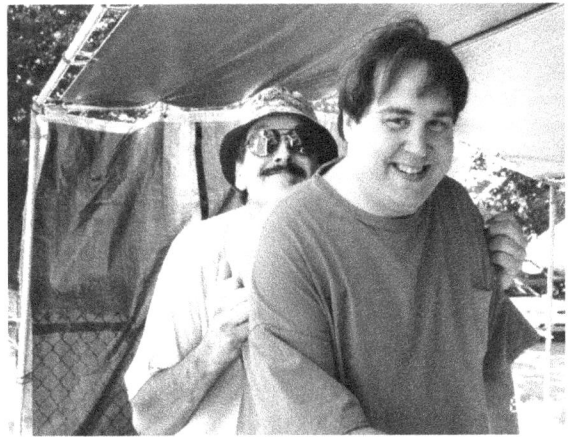

Raymond's brother Gerald. frying at an earlier fish fry. At rear is Pat Noland.

Behind him, inside the doorway another tall man, dark haired, in polo shirt and shorts, looks down, turns and with a slight hesitance, goes up the stairs. This is Raymond. He is the host of this party. He will likely spend most of it in front of his TV, on the couch, nursing a Pepsi.

Raymond has been working toward this fish fry for months. He set the date; he made up the guest list; he copied the invitations and helped send them out, hand delivering many of the cards. He made a big colorful fish poster to decorate the front of the house. He will spend some time eating crisp fish slices and potluck salads and sides with his guests and then retire to the safety and quiet of his living room, while they continue to party down on the lawn. Most of Raymond's guests are members of the ongoing "Futures Planning"* support group that Raymond and his family have pulled together over time to serve as his creative backup to support the many changes that have occurred for him.

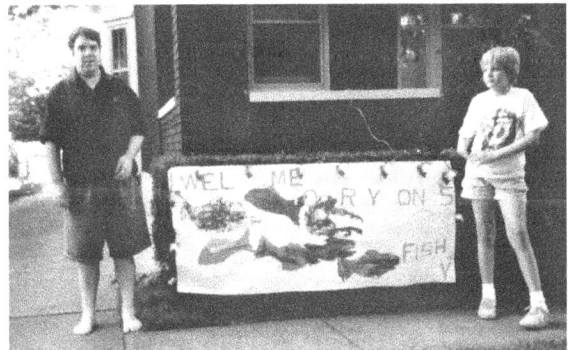

Raymond with his niece Mari Elizabeth Stansbury and a banner he made with Julie Cole.

*Indicates term in Glossary, page 139

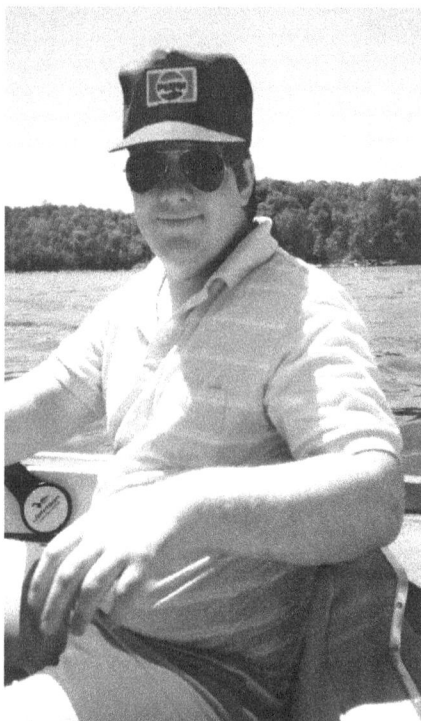

Raymond driving the boat on a fishing trip at Lake Cumberland.

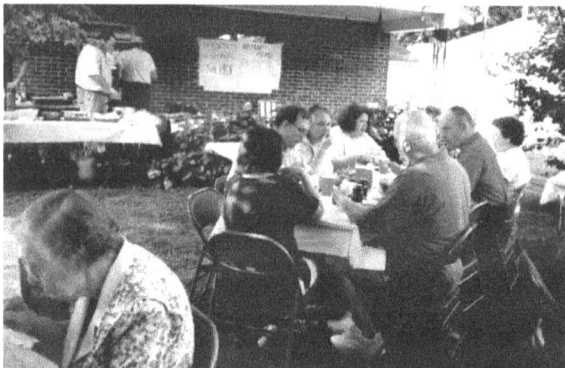

Enjoying the fish fry are, in front, Raymond's grandmother Christine Kandler, and around the table from left: Carolyn Wheeler, Tim Estes, Nancy Brucchieri, Linda McCauliffe, Ann Dittmeier, Clinton Montgomery, and Toby Wheeler.

Not your usual gracious host? Well, this is Raymond. He is a gracious host, but his unique personality makes his way of giving a party different from most. From birth he has related to people around him with difficulty. Speech came slowly for Raymond. Communication and comprehension always seemed somewhat limited for him as he matured. He didn't walk at the usual age and has had a lifelong mild motor deficit. Raymond's biggest barrier to being "usual" is an intense anxiety which he can't describe or explain. At times it leaks out of him with extreme energy, causing explosive bursts that often involve "moving" furniture, TVs, walls and doors as he tries unsuccessfully to express his rage and fears. When Raymond relaxes and is at his best, he is a man of quiet charm and good humor and is carefully affectionate with good friends. But he is still extremely shy and meets new people and situations with great trepidation.

This is his eighth fish fry, and many of his friends come to enjoy the family-caught fresh fish and Jennie's Moby Dick onion rings. But they mostly enjoy Raymond's company, and getting to know each other and each other's families better. They like to commiserate over the year past and how things in his life, and Raymond, have changed since Raymond's first fish fry.

The fish frys were originally Raymond's family's idea to share a good time with this emerging group of supporters for Raymond. The frys also extended Raymond's reach into his community. The first one celebrated Raymond's birthday in October, in the second year that the group had been meeting. Jim, Raymond's dad, and his buddy Arlen, and Carolyn and Denise, two of his four sisters, did all of the fishing for the frys and thus a tradition was born.

The reason for Raymond's group

Betty is Raymond's mother and the initial organizer of everything that happens for Raymond. It was her desperate need for more order and sanity in her home that made her reach out to others to find a bigger world for Raymond. She found Hope, and Jo Ann and the REACH* organization, and her support group all grew from that contact.

Along with the annual fish frys, the group held meetings either monthly or every six weeks, and smaller committee and focused-work gatherings were held as needed in between. Raymond's Futures Planning group had stayed together in a free-flowing, flexible way for nine years at the time of this fish fry. Betty, with Hope's help, made up her group with family, friends, neighbors, and local and statewide professionals in disability work. All but about six core members and family flowed in and out of the loosely-organized circle as they were needed, or felt able to contribute. What motivated these people to stay connected in support of this one man?

Tim Estes, one of the original group members says, "It's almost like there was an unconscious social organizing going on that centered around knowing Raymond as a human being, not a bundle of problems. This meant a great deal in the quality of his life. Raymond's success was being known as a human being."

Raymond's close and fiercely loyal family members, Betty and Jim, Denise, Dana, Donna, Carolyn, and Gerald were the backbone of the group. They reinforced successes that Raymond achieved. Their deep love for Raymond inspired others to see his inherently lovable nature.

Even when group members left due to job or location changes, or their roles changed in relation to Raymond, they usually stayed in touch and kept up with what was happening in Raymond's life.

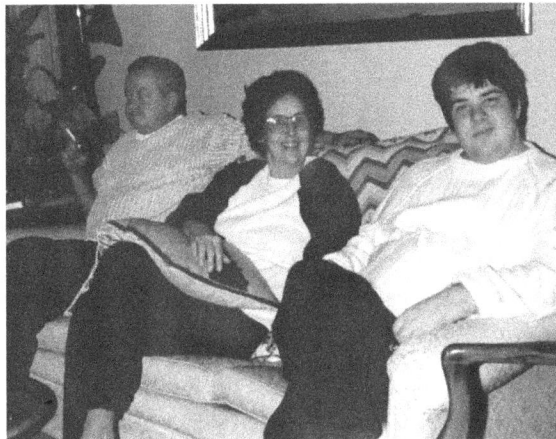

Raymond with mom Betty and dad Jim.

There was another component to this group that was a bit different from the usual support circle. As Milton Tyree, disability employment specialist and original member of Raymond's group, notes, "One of the things I think is different from other groups I have been in is that Raymond's group has a pretty high concentration of human service professionals. But I always felt that Raymond's group was involved because of our personal, not our professional identities."

These members, especially Milton Tyree, Nancy Brucchieri, Hope Dittmeier, Jo Ann Boyle, Tim Estes, Linda McAuliffe, Cindy Bayes, and later Carolyn Wheeler and Julie Cole, started out in "professional roles" with Raymond, and stayed, as Milton said, "personally." There were many other professionals invited by these members who were able to offer expertise and services. They came, some often, some only once, and several stayed in touch with the group in one way or another. Other professionals who supported Raymond and belonged to his group included Jim Schrecker, Owen and Julie McWilliams, Rocky Robinson, Gwen Harbuck, Lee Bobzien, Barry Whaley, Sally Shaikun, Becca Krall, Sarah Tackett, and a number of others who attended meetings as part of their roles with Raymond's day. All of their contributions were truly valuable. They often moved things along for Raymond with the various agencies that served him.

There were over 62 formal meetings recorded over the ten years, and often several meetings of little task groups between them. Most of the meetings were attended by eight to twelve people who, in the early years, gathered in Betty's bay-windowed dining room around the big table. Around 54 different people attended the recorded meetings at least one time.

They came in celebration of that community building around Raymond. It was probably from Betty that Raymond learned to be a generous host to all of his new friends. Even with Raymond's occasional uncomfortable behaviors, Betty had an open-door policy in her home. She made her home a place that others would want to come to. And to her home we came.

Raymond's history and childhood medical issues

Raymond was born October 4, 1966, the youngest of six. He was a handsome child with a thatch of dark hair. But he had a distant look in his eyes. Betty noticed him turning his head and eyes strongly to the left and staring up. "By the time he was six weeks old he was doing that a lot," Betty remembers. He was having multiple seizures.

Carolyn, his sister, recalls watching Raymond as she played and counting the times he'd have a seizure in order to help her mother keep track of the pattern. She didn't remember this as an unusual thing for a child to do because it was just what she did for her little brother.

Betty was referred by the pediatrician to Dr. Roth, a tall, lean man wearing black-rimmed glasses. He would be Raymond's neurologist and strong support for the family for years to come. Betty liked him for his laid-back attitude and consistent response to her concerns.

Raymond spent a lot of his first three years in hospitals because of the chronic seizures and repeated bouts of pneumonia. At home Betty rigged up a playpen with plastic covers to make an oxygen tent. Four times a day Raymond would be put in the tent for breathing treatments.

During one of these terrifying struggles with pneumonia, Betty bundled up the two-year-old Raymond and ran to the pediatrician she had been referred to. The doctor told Betty that he didn't think Raymond had pneumonia.

"I think he has pneumonia," Betty insisted. The doctor said, "What if I say he doesn't?"

Later, recalling the incident, Betty says, "Well, I told him I think that he does. He said he doesn't. I took Raymond home and bad went to worse. I called Dr. Roth, his neurologist, nearly every day. I told him, 'He is dying. He is the sickest boy I have ever seen.' Then he said, 'Bring the baby in.'

"When Dr. Roth saw Raymond, he was horrified. Raymond did in fact have bilateral pneumonia. He was so sick and hurting so much you couldn't touch him any where on his body that he didn't scream out in pain.

"'Oh my God, take him right over to St. Joe's,' Dr. Roth ordered. He called the pediatrician in to the hospital, and they worked over Raymond for a long time to get him back.

"When the baby got well Dr. Roth said, 'Don't take him back to that doctor.'"

Betty found another pediatrician for Raymond. He put Raymond in isolation for six weeks. He said that was to give Betty a rest. Betty remembers that as a horrible time.

"A nurse brought the baby to me saying she feared he was losing the will to live. I'll never forget how he held onto me tightly for two hours.

"That pediatrician seemed indifferent," she said.

"When Raymond was over three Dr. Roth said his tonsils should come out. Four doctors refused to do the surgery, fearing that Raymond wouldn't make it. Dr. Roth found a doctor who would do it, if Roth was in surgery with him. After that operation the pneumonia stopped.

"But in a little while that doctor sent me a letter saying he was referring me to another doctor. So we went to a third pediatrician, who said 'What is sad about this is these kids are only alive because of modern medicine but once they get past the age of three they live on, and who's to say that is the right thing to do?'

"Well, I don't know what I was supposed to say to that." Betty recalls angrily.

After that Dr. Roth said he would personally check on Raymond's physical condition, instead of calling in a pediatrician. Betty would call Dr. Roth, and if Raymond needed something extra he'd refer Betty to a specialist.

Family life and school experiences

A little ten-year-old curls up beside her toddler brother on his bed. He is not able to sleep and cries anxiously. She takes his hand and he grips her arm and holds tight. After a while he is breathing better and more regularly and not sobbing. She hopes he is asleep and quietly slides her arm out from under his. She wants to get to her bed to sleep. Just as her hand slips below his arm he grasps her hand and pulls her back down. She sighs, curls back close, and stays.

Because of his health struggles and the persistent seizures, Raymond's development was delayed, and his behaviors were often difficult. He would cry and throw things when he couldn't be understood. His first clear words were, "I love you," echoed to his mother when he was three. He didn't speak clearly again until at four he said "kitty cat."

He had trouble getting to sleep and Carolyn, six years older, would "buddy him" by staying with him until she thought he'd gone to sleep.

"Raymond sat up like most babies," Betty says. "But he didn't crawl until eighteen months. He inched along like an inchworm. When he was about five he would pull himself up to the sofa. I would kid him and tell him to back up. One day he did back up. I can still remember his giggle. So he walked backward before he walked forward. Then he took off."

At home his four sisters would play with Raymond while teaching him. They made up a circle game with Raymond in the middle. They would repeat a word, or a skill, like drinking through a straw. When he succeeded the girls would all bow and call him King Farouk. He would wave his hands and giggle at them. They also liked to tease him with names like "Fruita the Cockatiel." He didn't mind. He would repeat after them. Raymond also learned the cadences of favorite nursery rhymes. Years later he would incorporate some of these verses into his poems.

He got to be a crack shot at basketball by modeling his brother and sisters. They often included Raymond in their backyard ball games.

Raymond wanted to start school like his older siblings, proud to carry his pencil box and notebooks. But there were no specific programs for kids with disabilities in the public schools in Raymond's home town of Louisville, Ky., so he started out at the Stevens School, a residential school program for children with disabilities in Frankfort, Ky., about 50 miles away. Betty liked Raymond's teacher there, and no one told Betty of behavior problems.

Later, when the Louisville public schools began to accept children with disabilities, Raymond went to Henry Clay Elementary. The administration sent a lady to see the Athertons because the school staff believed Raymond couldn't walk. While she was at the house he went out the back door and down the steps. "Well, he will walk tomorrow," the teacher insisted.

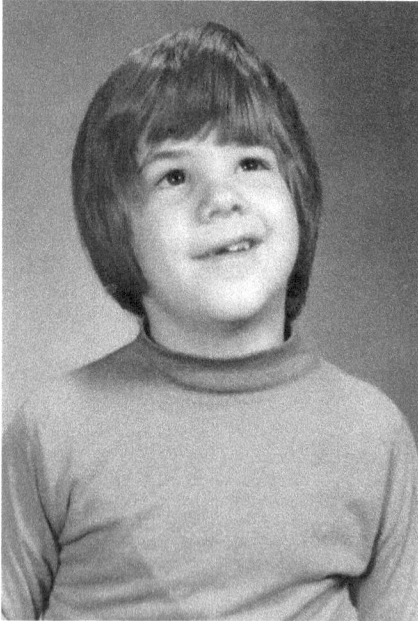

Raymond at six.

While Raymond attended Henry Clay his bus driver became a good friend. One day when Raymond refused to put on new shoes, Mr. English, the driver, took the shoes and Raymond. When Raymond got home he was wearing his shoes comfortably. Mr. English even stepped in to support Raymond when the principal refused to let Raymond go on field trips. The kind bus driver would assure the school that he would supervise Raymond on the trips. Despite these successes, the principal believed that Raymond didn't belong in that school.

Raymond was sent to the TIPP* program. It was a brief-duration residential program for children with behavior problems run by River Region, a regional program of federally-funded mental-health/mental-retardation services (now called Seven Counties Services*).

"This program was really successful for Raymond," Betty says. "He was home for weekends, but when we took him back he would jump out of the car and run to be with the TIPP staff and residents. He was happy there. They wanted to keep him longer, but you could only do one 'stint.'"

Raymond did his next "stint" at Churchill Park, a segregated school for disabled children. Betty feels that this placement was the start of Raymond's "real acting out." He had cried and shouted before, but the destructive episodes really started there. Betty remembers the principal telling the family that the way they had raised Raymond was the cause of his problems, and only they could change him.

"He also told us that Raymond was the only child in the county that acted that way.

That was difficult for me. I did a lot of thinking about where I had gone wrong, and how I had let Raymond down."

He was placed in a behaviorally disabled group, "a closed classroom" at Booker T. Washington Elementary. That just made things worse as he learned new and more difficult behaviors from other disturbed youngsters. Then he was sent to Tulley School, which was also a segregated public school for children with disabilities.

Betty recalls sending Raymond on the school bus with her heart in her throat.

"Raymond would break out one window on the school bus over and over. The teacher would call home after Raymond arrived at school and defend Raymond, 'It's the bus driver's fault; Raymond was being good. It was the bus driver.'

"The bus driver got tired of having broken windows. So finally a man came and drove Raymond to school personally.

"The next year the new teacher would call and complain about Raymond's acting out. And she went bananas."

Raymond's sister Carolyn remembers, "Mom and I went one day to Tulley School when they called Mom in. It was surprising to see Raymond in that setting. He didn't look like the Raymond we knew at home. He took on looks and traits like the other children at the school. Obviously he wasn't happy there and they weren't happy having him there. They didn't know how to communicate with him or how to treat him. There was a lot of frustration on both sides."

Raymond's brother Gerald adds, "That's when I felt they were warehousing people with disabilities in the schools. I don't remember much of his school years day-to-day, but I remember the outcomes. Looking back I realize how much Raymond copied others. He'd come home with his arm all drawn up. He was emulating the other kids. He would do things or act in ways that he saw the other kids do. Right then the teachers should have listened to Mom when she told them, 'He's not like that at home.'"

At Tulley School one teacher, Ms. Accordino, saw potential in Raymond. She was careful and persistent in her attempts to help him learn to read. He enjoyed working with her and grew to trust her. They worked together happily. But after his successful year with her, things deteriorated.

Each school would send a letter to the family requesting that he not be sent back. Home tutoring was not successful in his middle school years. Betty would take Raymond to Doctor Roth when he was taken out of schools. The doctor would say that it was the school's problem that they couldn't meet Raymond's needs. This just led to Betty deciding that it wasn't worth the hassle to try to send Raymond back to school. Yet she feared the schools would sue her for his truancy. Dr. Roth said, "Keep him home. By the time they get around to suing you, he will be over sixteen."

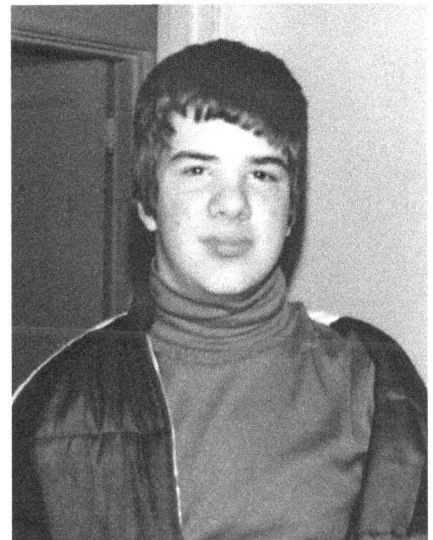

Raymond at thirteen.

Raymond's behavioral issues were getting more serious as he grew older. Betty made repeated requests for some kind of help, some support for the family because of Raymond's increasing anxiety and physical acting out. During Raymond's late teens and into his twenties, she asked for assistance from Seven Counties Services, the regional comprehensive care center. They didn't seem to be able to offer Betty any support at that time for Raymond; instead, they referred her for psychiatric help.

In his mid-twenties Raymond began to use lithium prescribed by Dr. Roth to stabilize his mood. He also took Haldol* to slow down what had become rapid bursts of shouting, and a need to "move furniture," as Raymond described it.

Raymond was in his twenties. He spent his time at home with Betty. Occasionally he'd go on errands with Betty to the store, or to family medical appointments. Sometimes they would visit Raymond's grandparents or Betty's friends. Like any guy his age living with his parents with no job or place to go during the day, Raymond was probably bored. He had no way to tell others about this; his conversation was limited, practical, demanding, and often echolalic. He'd repeat questions to people over and over, but was able to answer only very simple questions directed at him. Most of the time he sat in front of the TV with the remote control in his hand.

Like other men his age, Raymond might have wanted to leave his parents' home. His family believed he would be unable to leave home due to his mental disability, his debilitating fears in public places, and his loud, explosive, and sometimes damaging reactions to stressful circumstances. So part of Raymond may have been angry about being stuck at home, while another part of him didn't want to leave home. This possible internal conflict may have added to Raymond's chronic anxiety. Since he couldn't express this to anyone, no one could really know.

Raymond's dad, Jim, was coming to the end of his rope. Raymond would try to get him to stay home from work. Betty felt that Raymond's urgent need for his parents to stay at home with him might have started since his brother and sisters had all left home. Jim had to convince Raymond that he had to leave for work and that he would be home later and would not go away.

Betty was chronically exhausted and stressed. She would get relief from Raymond's constant presence and persistent needs and demands by going out into the back yard, where he could see her from the family room. There she would dig dandelions and violets from the lawn, until he called her back in. Sometimes she'd escape to the basement to do laundry, but if she stayed too long Raymond would be at the top of the stairs yelling for her to come back up.

His sister Denise was worried for her parents' health. She began talking about institutions.

"Raymond had been an unusual child," Betty tells us. "But I was optimistic and hopeful for his future despite his school problems and health issues, until he was about fifteen years old. Then I became really worried. In his teen years, Raymond's behaviors had become so bizarre that I was totally frustrated and didn't see much of a future for him."

So Betty's life was tightly compressed by her wish to support Raymond in his own home. Her husband wasn't able to cope as well with Raymond's requirements for routine, sameness, control, and his need to shout out spontaneously to relieve stress and to "move furniture," suddenly through the air, when his anxiety level would peak.

Jim sought solitude and often withdrew from Raymond and Betty. Betty would encourage him to take weekend fishing trips. "There was no sense in two of us being confined to the house.

"Our adult children were the only support we had had over those years," Betty would say. But at this crisis time, his siblings all lived away, in California, Nebraska, and Indiana.

What to do next?

"When Raymond was in a really bad cycle and his behaviors were most distressing and out of control, I called Seven Counties Services again and begged for help," Betty recalls.

"I called everyone in the state capital, Frankfort, at every agency I could think of. We got no response. I felt like I had gotten to the bottom of a black hole.

"That was when I was invited to attend a parent respite information group. I disrupted every meeting until they asked if I would like to go to the REACH seminar. At the meeting I found out what REACH was from what the speaker said, and from a brochure that I picked up.

"It said, 'Resources for Education, Adaptation, Change, and Health, Inc. is a program set up to provide person-centered planning for families with disabled or disturbed children.

"'The organization has evolved from a home-visiting psychology practice to a comprehensive support system for families (including foster families) with difficult-to-serve individuals. Direct services provided include therapeutic foster care, respite, crisis prevention and intervention, school consultation, recreational programming, and interagency collaboration and planning.'

"Later I found out that REACH had developed a grant program called Outreach, 'To find several families in the Commonwealth and support those families in innovative ways as they made decisions about life goals for their children with disabilities.' (www.reachoflouisville.com)

"At the REACH seminar I spoke to everyone I came in contact with about how bad things had become at home. I met and sat down to lunch with Jo Ann Boyle, a young facilitator from REACH. She listened politely to my desperate story and asked a few questions. After I left I didn't give it any more thought. It would be just another dead end."

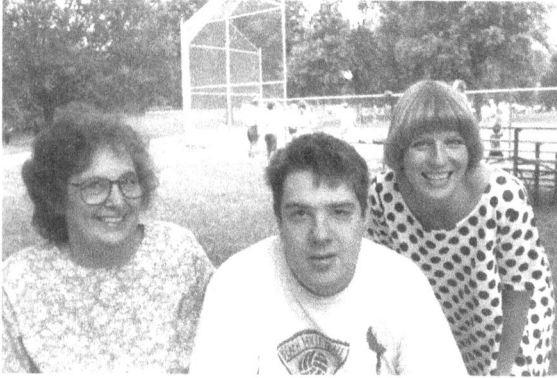

Jo Ann Boyle, right, with Betty and Raymond.

Jo Ann recalls, "I explained to Betty what we could offer Raymond through the grant at our luncheon meeting. I remember she was somewhat hesitant, only because what she had been promised in the past had never happened. She agreed to let us contact her in the future."

Betty continues, "Well, she called the next day and said she didn't know if she could help but that she would like to try. She said she had to talk to Hope Dittmeier, who was in charge of this Outreach program. I was doubtful, but I thanked her and saw a little ray of light as I said I'd look forward to her call."

Jo Ann remembers, "I offered to help Betty without discussing any of this with Hope or Bob Ilback, the creators of the grant. I was acting somewhat outside of my authority. When I spoke to Hope, she initially was not willing to become involved, only because it sounded like an impossible situation. We wanted to be set up for some degree of success. With a little thought, or perhaps because I confessed that I had already offered our help, Hope agreed to allow us to become involved with Raymond, if Raymond was willing."

Hope describes her side of the contact. Jo Ann came to her with the desperate story she heard from a gracious but stressed-out mother.

"I think Jo Ann Boyle deserves a tremendous amount of credit. She was very skilled. But she didn't have a lot of experience. She was courageous. She came to me saying, 'I'd like to do this.' I said, 'Jo Ann, are you sure you are not getting in over your head? I am not going to tell you no.' I trusted her judgment. She was smart enough to set up some safeguards for herself."

"Jo Ann called Betty back and talked with her about what she was going to do to get things rolling. She explained to Betty, "The Outreach grant from the Developmental Disabilities Council was designed to offer people with disabilities an opportunity to live in the community that is not possible under the current options."

Jo Ann said, "We considered alternative possibilities for individuals with a process called 'Personal Futures Planning.' The process involves the person with the disability and a group of people who get to know the person well. That group then works to creatively develop ideas to make the 'focus' person's dreams and desires come true."

First Jo Ann met with Betty and Raymond together to ask a lot of questions in order to build graphic maps of his life and his dreams. They talked for quite a while so that Jo Ann would have a history of Raymond's life, and ideas of the scope of his current life and activities. She would then construct a visual map of his current situation on large paper which could be added to by the group of friends invited to Raymond's first Futures Planning meeting.

Jo Ann looks back at that very first encounter with Raymond. "I'm not really sure why everything worked out, but I do remember meeting with Betty and being introduced to Raymond for the first time. He was sitting on a couch, clothed in sweat clothes, barefoot, with a remote control in his hand, diligently watching TV. Betty and I held our meeting at a table a few feet away, where Raymond could eavesdrop on our conversation. I don't remember Raymond's reaction to my presence, but I remember that I was prepared to experience the worst from Raymond. It was clear that I made him nervous, but Betty graciously kept Raymond's apprehension settled while she shared his life story with me. It was a story of fitting a round block in a square hole, and blaming the ill fit on the block. Raymond was never offered a fair chance in a streamlined system, and he was smart enough to realize it and give the world grief for it. Good for him. As a result, public education didn't work for him, public services didn't work for him, but he had a family that loved him, believed in him, and treated him with respect."

Raymond agreed to have a meeting in the community clubhouse, with some of his closest and his newest friends invited.

So with a new set of maps and his history ready, and the right people invited, and Raymond's permission, Jo Ann and Betty set a date for the initial meeting.

Circle Origins – REACH and the Dream

"That first meeting was held on October 17, 1991," Jo Ann remembers, "and included Betty, who was hostess; Raymond, who wasn't too sure about being there; Jennie Needy, a neighbor and friend of Betty; Dana Atherton, one of Raymond's sisters; Lucy Axton, an advisor from Seven Counties who specialized in creative employment and funding; Tim Estes, also then at Seven Counties; Milton Tyree, who was then with an agency which developed employment for people with disabilities; Hope Dittmeier, and Jo Ann Boyle, with REACH."

Betty recalls, "We had our first meeting at the community center because we were unsure how Ray would handle a lot of people at home, some who were friends, but others who were new. Jo Ann and Hope had asked most of the group to come, and I asked Dana and Jennie.

"Jo Ann Boyle outlined Raymond's life in words and pictures on large paper "maps" hung around the room. It had gotten to the point that I could only picture an institution

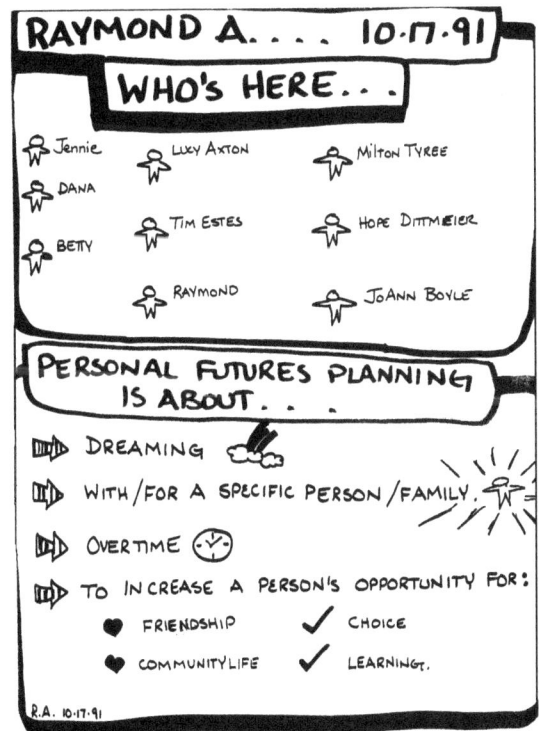

RAYMOND A. . . . 10·17·91
WHO'S HERE. . . .

Jennie   Lucy Axton   Milton Tyree
Dana
Betty   Tim Estes   Hope Dittmeier

             Raymond   JoAnn Boyle

PERSONAL FUTURES PLANNING IS ABOUT. . . .

➭ DREAMING
➭ WITH/FOR A SPECIFIC PERSON/FAMILY.
➭ OVERTIME
➭ TO INCREASE A PERSON'S OPPORTUNITY FOR:
   ♥ FRIENDSHIP   ✓ CHOICE
   ♥ COMMUNITY LIFE   ✓ LEARNING.

R.A. 10·17·91

for the rest of Raymond's days, but Jo Ann would say quietly, 'We don't believe in that, and we will work hard to figure out another way.'"

Jo Ann Boyle describes the experience as not the usual support meeting.

"The thing that I was most moved about at this meeting was the energy and fun that the family had put into planning the meeting. A wonderful spread of food and drink was provided, and Raymond was, without a doubt, the man of the moment. We reviewed his life story. Raymond was wonderfully honest throughout the telling of his story.

"When we came across a point in his life that was somewhat painful, he would scream out with a deep, loud sound that would knock your socks off. 'No!!' It shook my bones apart each time. This was a young man who had a keen way of feeling and sharing his experiences, rather than just living them. Things that had happened years before still left him raw with emotions."

Hope recalls, "I don't know many facilitators who could have handled that first meeting as she did. With Raymond's screaming, she was afraid; a number of us in that room were afraid.

"If you look in the minutes and the notes, it is clear what the dream was. She hit it right on the head to begin with. It was a dream of a place for Raymond in the community, with a home, and work, and friends, and a good life. With skill and enthusiasm, Jo Ann got the right people to the table and established enough rapport with Raymond for him to let her do this. She deserves a lot of credit."

From that initial meeting, it all began.

A Raymond Poem

July 14, 1997

...I was packing the cooler. Soft drinks in the cooler.

Beer in the cooler. Root beer in the cooler.

Watermelon beer. Fruit pie. Watermelon beer.

No, Dad went fishing. I don't know.

Carolyn caught crappie. Two bass. One crappie.

Daddy cleaned them.

Snailsoup, peanut butter.

What's wrong with you Julie, Pencil.

Exclamation point!!!!!!

I am running around. I went HQ

Water glasses at HQ.

Macaroni dish. Jim's gonna make it.

Julie is bringing broccoli casserole.

Nancy is bringing carrots with a spoon.

Carolyn is going to, no Dana is bringing dip.

Milton is going to bring cantaloupe.

Jennie will bring pizza rolls.

Denise and Pat are coming. I don't know what they'll bring.

Cupcakes, maybe pizza pie.

Gerald is coming, my Gerald. He'll bring more carrots.

Mom is cooking raspberries and a can of beans.

Linda is coming. She might bring a cake, and a casserole.

Hope will bring marshmallows.

Raspberry pie, Linda does those.

The fish fry is August 23rd. At 8:00 p.m.

Evening time.

It is going to be fun.

There will be Pepsi, root beer, lemonade, pretzels.

Chip dip. Dana is bringing that.

Paper plates. She's going to get a kick out of it.

Macaroni party. Jim fixes that.

Meemaw's coming. She'll fix tato salad.

It's a pizza party. At my place.

Raspberries.

Back to the fish fry

The breeze is a little cooler, and the dusk is deeper and the fryer is off. The tables are still filled with guests nibbling fancy frosting from Linda's cupcakes, or washing one of Julie's kitchen-sink cookies down with cold soda. The light is on in the little triangular gable which fronts Raymond's upstairs bedroom.

Milton and Vicky are talking with Nancy and Jennie while watching their daughter play near the porch.

"It has been an amazing year. It's still hard to believe Raymond's here in his duplex. He really seems to be loving it." Nancy fans herself with a loose paper plate.

"He stayed out for quite a while tonight."

"Who wouldn't? The food was great." Julie pulls out the chair next to Nancy and plops down.

"It has been a remarkable year," Milton says, bending to fix Kaylyn's shoe strap. "Carolyn and Syd and Betty really deserve the credit for pulling off this whole house purchase and renovation."

"And Hope, too. She jumpstarted things and got 'em moving. And then she takes off for Wisconsin. I hated that." Nancy smiles regretfully.

Linda sits down next to her with a glass of tea. "Leaving us with the persistent problem of finding Raymond a few good people to help build his day. Recruitment is such a struggle. It was hard enough finding Raymond a roommate. I am sorry Tony didn't work out, but we knew what we were getting into, kind of. Now Raymond has Bryan and his dogs." Linda fans herself with a spare paper plate.

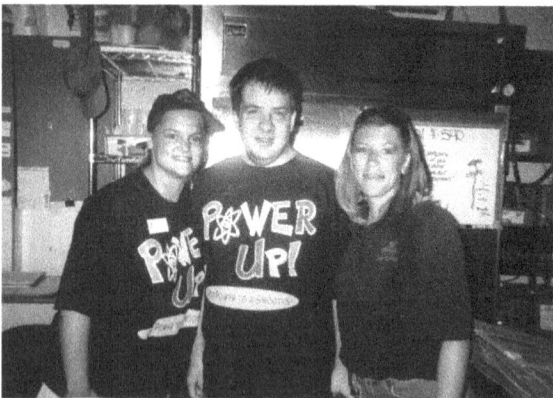
Raymond with co-workers at Frulatti's.

Milton sips soda, as the light continues to fade. "I bet Raymond would like to be able to go back to Frulatti's to work like he did with Pat. At least he still has his church bulletins job that Nancy found for him."

"It's hard to realize how sick Pat has gotten. Betty and Raymond have been visiting him every week at Mt. Holly. She says he's not doing very well." Nancy leans into the paper table cover where her Sprite has left a puddle of condensation. Jennie nods her head. Pat, Raymond's sister Denise's friend, had been Raymond's day program* companion for some time. He would spend time each day with Raymond, planning activities and taking Raymond to do interesting and productive things. Raymond was enjoying their time together, especially his part-time job at Frulatti's, a little café in the food court at the Mall. He got a kick out of putting cookies on baking trays. preparing fruit for salads. and the camaraderie of the little store's staff.

"At the next meeting we'll have to ask each person to take and hand out some of the recruitment ads that Hope wrote and Gerald updated. We all have all kinds of contacts; we just have to push them more, to find other day companions for Raymond." Nancy laughs.

"Who should we focus on?" Julie mumbles through a chocolate brownie.

"We need to find people who affect Raymond like Gerald does," Nancy muses. She is one of the easy-going people that Raymond really enjoys spending time with.

"Raymond likes people who help him feel safe and comfortable. Jim Schrecker and Owen McWilliams have been good companions for Raymond. They are large, flexible, fairly laid-back presences who Raymond relates to well, for the most part."

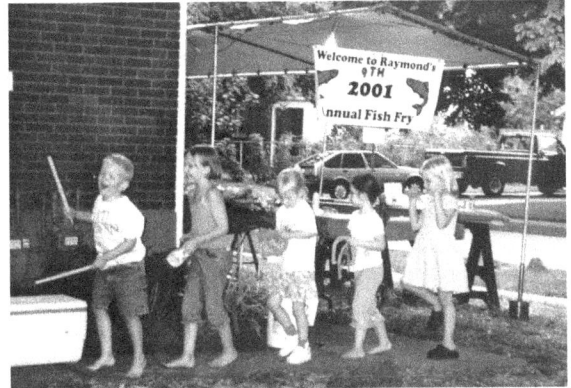

Children open a fish fry with a parade.

Milton and Vicky's Kaylyn wanders back to ask Vicky a question.

"I am going in to say goodnight to Raymond. Got an early meeting in Lexington in the morning." Nancy smiles at everyone as she heads into the house.

Millie Comp from Disability Court is talking with Gwen Harbuck, who had been Raymond's program coordinator* from Seven Counties Services, about Gwen's change of job, and her move to the country. Linda McAuliffe puts the last few cupcakes in her cardboard bakery box. Gerald, Syd, and Carolyn are taking pans in from the fry area.

"One more bite? You don't want it to go to waste." Tim Estes declines Betty's joking offer. Carol urges him to get ready to make the long trip back home to Warsaw, Kentucky. She knows he has things to do before he leads church services in the morning. Carolyn and Toby Wheeler make their farewells to Betty and the gang and set out for Lexington.

The lawn is nearly empty now and the street lights and the parking lot lights from the two big churches across the street shine just enough for dawdling guests not to trip on oak tree roots near the tables as the last few cars start to pull away.

Raymond is on his sofa watching the evening news. Gerald has his feet up watching with him.

Chapter 2

The Methods of the Circle

Futures planning

When Jo Ann Boyle met Betty at the REACH conference they began a process that is becoming a model for support for people with disabilities living in communities all over the country. Betty was not aware that such an idea was growing, but she became a willing participant in a movement full of energy and hope.

REACH was using a concept and model called "Personal Futures Planning."

Hope Dittmeier, Jo Ann Boyle's supervisor from REACH, was involved in the concept very early in Kentucky.

Hope describes it this way:

> Person-centered planning is not just a trendy technique or method. It is an approach; a way to go about determining and implementing ways to support a particular individual. It involves a group of concerned people who come together and are encouraged to understand the "focus person" in a way that promotes that person's contributions, choices, and control.

> Person-centered planning is not value-neutral. The process embraces a set of values or principles that define what quality of life means. John O'Brien's five accomplishments describe it best:

> **Community Presence** – How can we increase the presence of a person in local community life?

> **Community Participation** – How can we expand and deepen people's friendships?

> **Encouraging Valued Social Roles** – How can we enhance the reputation people have and increase the number of valued ways people can contribute?

> **Promoting Choice** – How can we help people have more control and choice in life?

> **Supporting Contribution** – How can we assist people to develop more competencies?

There are a variety of tools designed to implement person-centered planning. Marsha Forest and Jack Pearpoint developed the MAPS process; Beth Mount created Personal Futures Planning; Michael Smull produced Essential Lifestyle Planning; and John O'Brien created the PATH method [See bibliography, page 137]. What all these tools or techniques have in common is the commitment to the values mentioned above in the "Five Accomplishments." In Raymond's situation, we used Personal Futures Planning, primarily because it was best known by the facilitators.

Person-centered planning relies heavily on investing the time and energy to get to know and understand the focus person before decisions are made. It is critical that the person has a majority voice in the process. Person Centered Planning calls us to learn to listen to people more than we have ever done before. Some people are very articulate and can tell you clearly what their dreams and desires are. Others have more subtle or confusing ways of communicating. Our listening might include attending to the words, gestures and behavior of the focus person. In Raymond's situation, this meant watching for big smiles and honoring the loud "NO's."

Profile Maps

To initiate the Personal Futures Planning process the facilitator first meets the focus person and his/her family. Explaining how the process unfolds so that the focus person and the family are aware of the challenges, risks, and commitment involved is an important first step. Once the decision to proceed is made, the facilitator begins gathering Profile information about the focus person. This is generated by using "maps." Each map is a sheet of paper which portrays information about a particular area in colorful words and graphics. Maps include:

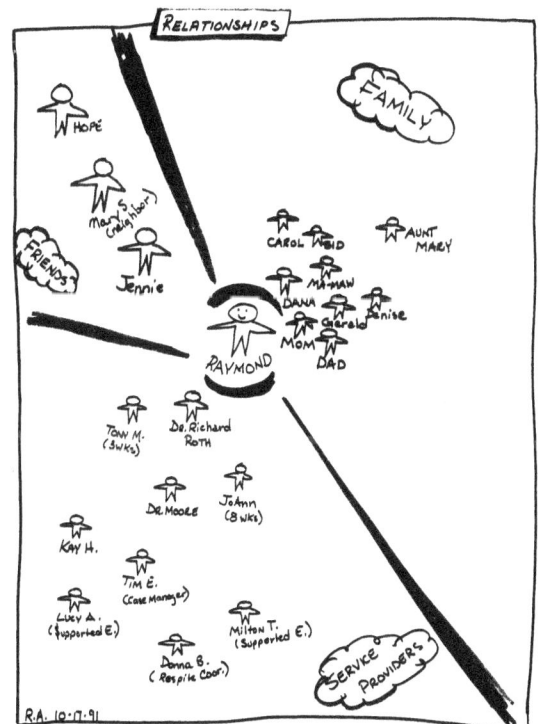

Relationships, including friends, family, and paid providers

Places in the community and human service world where the person spends time

Background history

Personal preferences, including what works and doesn't work for the person

Dreams, Hopes and Fears

Additional profile maps may be completed as deemed helpful, such as choices, daily routine, respect, communication, health, home, work. Most of this information

PLACES

MS. KATHEN Ice MNTH.

MA-MAW Ice WK.

DENICE Ice Month.

DANA Ice-4-6 WKS. IN/OUT Ice WK.

HOME — SPENDS 80% of HIS TIME AT HOME. DURING THE GOOD SIDE!

APPTS. DR. ROTH DR. MOORE

RUNS ERRANDS WITH MOM — KROGER — BUY-LOW — MALLS — BULL-FROG CREEK — MEANS DAD GOES FISHING!

R.A. 10·17·91

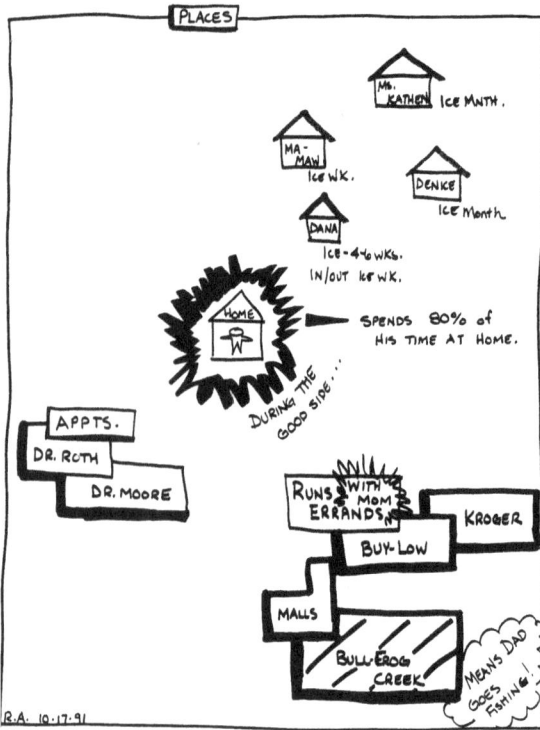

is gleaned from interviews with the focus person and the people who know her best. On rare occasions, a facilitator might refer to a service record for detail. While completing the profile, the facilitator strives to develop an honest, respectful, and trusting relationship with the focus person and their family.

Guest List

Once the Profile information is drafted, the facilitator, the focus person, and their family determine who they want to be involved in the process and a guest list is developed. The involvement of those who know and love the focus person best is critical. Often guest lists will include neighbors, friends, ministers, co-workers, or grandparents. Raymond's guest list was heavily weighted with people who knew him well – mom, sisters and brothers, and a life-long friend. His guest list also included human service professionals who were invited by the facilitator in hopes they might serve Raymond.

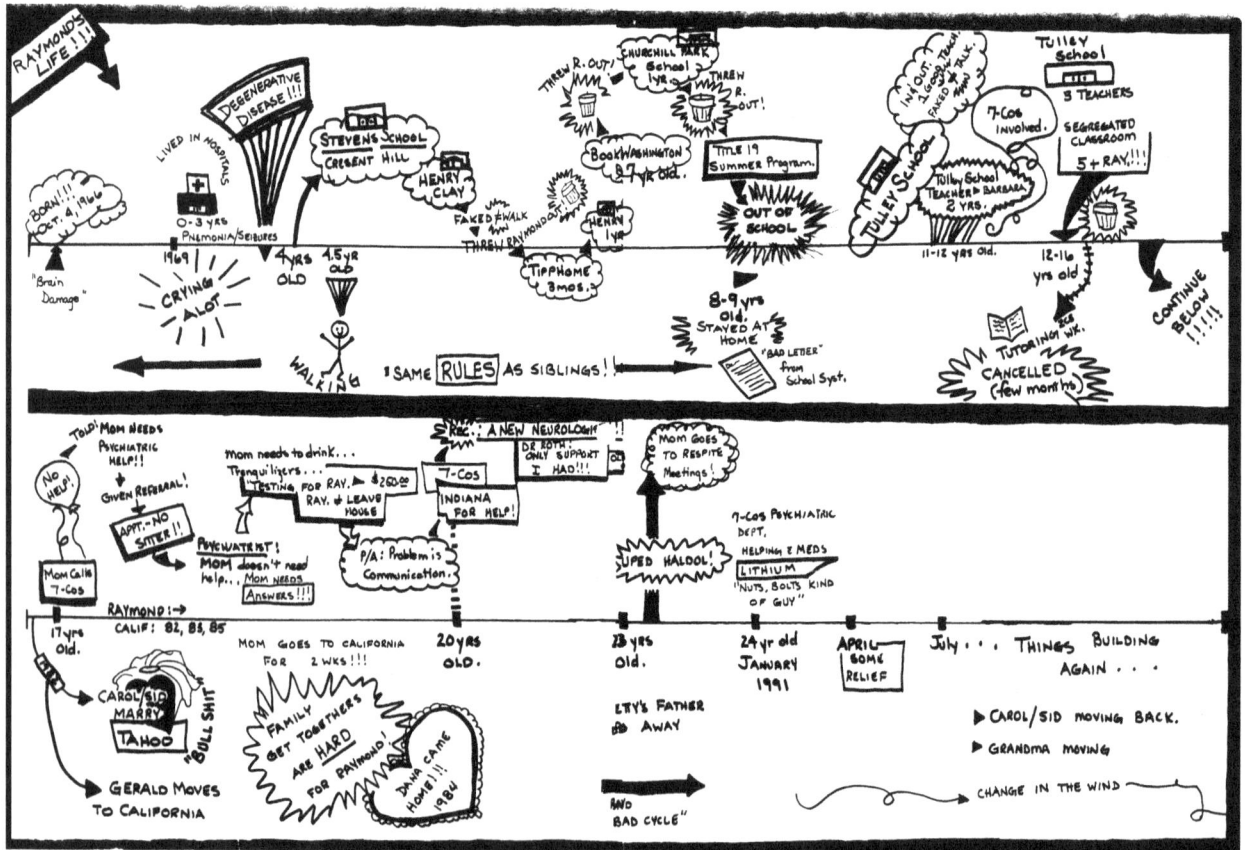

RAYMOND'S LIFE!!! — hand-drawn timeline of Raymond's life including: BORN!!! OCT. 4, 1966; "Brain Damage"; 0-3 YRS PNEUMONIA/SEIZURES; 1969 CRYING A LOT; LIVED IN HOSPITALS; DEGENERATIVE DISEASE!!!; STEVENS SCHOOL CRESENT HILL; HENRY CLAY; FAKED WALK; THREW RAYMOND OUT; 4 YRS OLD; 4.5 YR OLD; WALKING; SAME RULES AS SIBLINGS!; TIPP HOME 3 mos.; BOOKER WASHINGTON 6-7 YR OLD; THREW R. OUT!; CHURCHILL PARK School 1 yr; THREW R. OUT!; HENRY 1 yr; TITLE 19 Summer Program; OUT OF SCHOOL; 8-9 yrs old STAYED AT HOME; "BAD LETTER" from School Syst.; 11-12 yrs old; IN/OUT 1 GOOD TEACHER FAKED AGAIN; TULLEY School 3 TEACHERS; 7-COS involved; SEGREGATED CLASSROOM 5 + RAY!!!; TULLEY SCHOOL TEACHER BARBARA 3 YRS; 12-16 yrs old; TUTORING WK. CANCELLED (few months); CONTINUE BELOW!!!!; 17 yrs Old. RAYMOND → CALIF: '82, '83, '85; No HELP!; MOM CALLS 7-COS; Told: MOM NEEDS PSYCHIATRIC HELP!!; GIVEN REFERRAL!; APPT.—NO SITTER!!; PSYCHIATRIST! MOM doesn't need help... MOM NEEDS Answers!!!; Mom needs to drink... Tranquilizers... TESTING FOR RAY. & LEAVE HOUSE; P/A: Problem is Communication.; REC.: A NEW NEUROLOGIST; DR. ROTH: ONLY SUPPORT I HAD!!; 7-COS INDIANA FOR HELP!; Mom GOES TO RESPITE Meetings!; UPPED HALDOL!; 7-COS PSYCHIATRIC DEPT. HELPING & MEDS LITHIUM "NUTS, BOLTS KIND OF GUY"; CAROL/SID MARRY TAHOO; "BULL SHIT"; GERALD MOVES TO CALIFORNIA; MOM GOES TO CALIFORNIA FOR 2 WKS!!!; FAMILY GET TOGETHERS ARE HARD for Raymond!; DANA CAME HOME IN 1984 "AND BAD CYCLE"; 20 yrs OLD.; 23 yrs Old.; CITY'S FATHER IS AWAY; 24 yr old JANUARY 1991; APRIL SOME RELIEF; July... THINGS BUILDING AGAIN...; CAROL/SID moving BACK.; GRANDMA moving; CHANGE IN THE WIND

Location, Location, Location

Next, a place to convene the first meeting must be located. Often it is the person's home, a public library or community center meeting room, or a church classroom. Raymond and his family decided upon the nearby community center. The date and time of the meeting is dictated by the availability of those on the guest list, which may require evening or weekend times. Raymond's group, however, was available to meet in the afternoon. Finally, an invitation specifying the reason for meeting along with the date, time, and place is designed and distributed, requesting that guests RSVP.

Time

Typically a first meeting will last two hours. The meeting room is arranged in a casual, friendly circle and food and drink are served. The meeting begins with introductions. The Profile information is displayed on large pieces of paper, completed with colored markers. The facilitator reviews the Profile, asking participants to contribute any additional information or ask relevant questions. This process encourages the team to develop a common understanding and positive portrayal of the focus person.

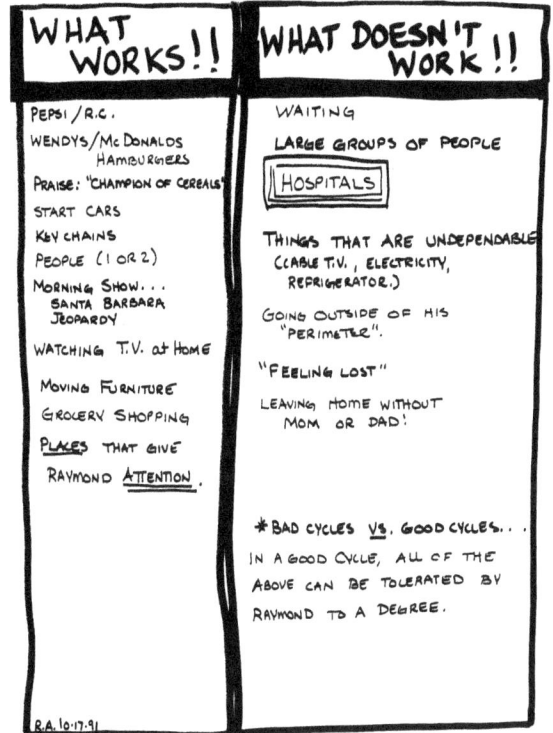

WHAT WORKS!!

PEPSI / R.C.
WENDYS / McDONALDS HAMBURGERS
Praise: "CHAMPION OF CEREALS"
START CARS
KEY CHAINS
PEOPLE (1 OR 2)
MORNING SHOW...
  SANTA BARBARA
  JEOPARDY
WATCHING T.V. at HOME
MOVING FURNITURE
GROCERY SHOPPING
PLACES THAT GIVE RAYMOND ATTENTION.

WHAT DOESN'T WORK!!

WAITING
LARGE GROUPS OF PEOPLE
HOSPITALS

THINGS THAT ARE UNDEPENDABLE (CABLE T.V., ELECTRICITY, REFRIGERATOR.)
GOING OUTSIDE OF HIS "PERIMETER".
"FEELING LOST"
LEAVING HOME WITHOUT MOM OR DAD!

* BAD CYCLES VS. GOOD CYCLES...
IN A GOOD CYCLE, ALL OF THE ABOVE CAN BE TOLERATED BY RAYMOND TO A DEGREE.

R.A. 10-17-91

Dreams

The group then develops an "image of a desirable future." The image describes a positive, typical lifestyle. It is a description of what the person's life would ideally be like, based on their unique interests and preferences. This typically will include the following:

Home – details about the type of housing desired (house, apartment, condo), the location of the home, and with whom the person would live, etc.

Work or school – details about what kind of work he prefers, what type of setting would most likely work for him, etc.

Social life – specifics about the new friendships she might like. What social and recreational activities she may want to get involved in, etc.

Person-centered planning teams aren't limited by what is currently offered by the human service system. The team will be creative in supporting a lifestyle that is an "ideal" imagined by and on behalf of the focus person. Instead of simply making referrals to residential programs, slots, or services, teams work to describe that ideal: a customized home setting. Rather than relying on established vocational options, teams describe desirable work or job training options. Without limiting the options for socialization to programs designed to serve people with disabilities, teams will look for ways to help the focus person develop new friendships, perhaps using the person's team members' network of friends. This was especially relevant for Raymond as there were no established programs willing and/or able to serve him. For the process to work for him, Raymond's supports were going to have to be custom-designed for him.

The team's future image will change and evolve over time. It is difficult in the beginning to describe a detailed futures map. Based on the circumstances, people may only be able to try to imagine the next step. This was the case in Raymond's story. "To have a bigger world" was as much as the team could initially see. Over time, that image became clearer – "To volunteer at Meals on Wheels" and later "To get a job at Frulatti's lunch diner." Other images over time included "To join the YMCA" and, "To have adult friends to hang out with on weekends," and finally, "To live in his own home!"

Action

Learning about the focus person and dreaming about a desirable future is usually quite enjoyable. The hard work starts when the desirable future is defined and the team is commissioned with finding out how to make it happen! Personal Futures Planning employs a problem-solving approach to action. The facilitator leads the group through a process where both community and service resources are identified, challenges are explored, solutions are considered, and action steps agreed upon. Through this process the members of the team determine how to proceed with developing support that is most meaningful to the focus person.

Funding

The availability of fiscal resources is often a challenge to teams. Sometimes a person has human service resources available for support, but the funds are not flexible enough to be utilized in unique ways. For instance, residential services are available if you are willing to live in an established group home owned and operated by an agency. Or, respite services are available as long as the agency has a provider willing to serve the person. Or, a person must receive eight hours of day programming each day, or none at all. These were just a small sample of the financial challenges Raymond and his Personal Futures Planning team had to address. [There is more information about the challenges of funding in Chapter 11.]

It happens, rarely, that a team meets a handful of times and is successful in creating the desirable future. On the other hand, it is also rare for a planning team to meet consistently over a ten-year period of time, as Raymond's group did. During much of those ten years, Raymond's team met monthly. There were times that subgroups of the team were meeting weekly, and there were periods of time when the group went six to eight weeks between meetings. The work of the group never seemed "finished."

Graphic facilitation*

From the first, Jo Ann Boyle incorporated the technique of Graphic Facilitation into the method of presentation in each meeting. The first meeting was on "neutral ground," in a neighborhood community room. Betty feared that Raymond would be more disruptive if the meeting was in his home. But meetings thereafter were held in Betty's dining room with its generous table, bright bay window, and mirrored sideboard, regularly crowded with circle members. The wall was festooned with sheets of newsprint or white poster paper, applied with masking tape. Carefully chosen non-permanent washable markers helped keep the pictures from bleeding onto the wall under the papers.

"Hello, everyone! Thanks for coming. You are all here at the top of the sheet." Jo Ann or Hope and later Tim, Nancy, Linda, or Carolyn would draw little figures for each person at the meeting, next to their names. Then the agenda for the meeting would be noted on the sheets, with lively pictures describing each item, and branches or webs connecting ideas with action steps and expected outcomes.

Graphic facilitation, as used by some of Raymond's group marker holders, is a method developed by David Sibbet and others to enhance a group's focus of attention, and potential for creative thought. Sibbet and a network of group process experts found, through years of experiential research, that groups using graphics retained information, felt more compelled to act on what was presented, and saw the organizing elements of the information more clearly and concisely.

"Drawings turned out to be magical and complex worlds with the potential to catalyze amazing insights during group process. They became a bridge to storytelling and other holistic mental practices." (The Grove Consultants International – www. grove.com)

Jack Pearpoint clarified for Betty and Julie later in a Path workshop the role that graphics play in the MAPS/Path process. When you draw a thought, not just write it out, it pulls you into a process which is not the usual way of thinking for most of us. It is not just "easier" to see the idea. The idea comes from and resonates with a different part of thinking, a part we are less apt to habitually use.

So if we jump out of our usual habits of thought and into new realms of creative process, it is likely we will link into and put forth new kinds of ideas. We can be cliché here about things like "thinking outside of the box," "lateral thinking," or we can draw up on that paper a picture of people crawling out of a hole onto a new planet, a place of brand new ways to look at things and create new paths for people. And we can move on from there.

Raymond's group started out with the pre-developed set of "maps," drawn up

SKILLS, GIFTS, & CONTRIBUTIONS

Good understanding on Electronic thing's!

EXCELLENT VOCABULARY

Makes needs Known.

Self-hygiene skills

Can ask for HELP when needed

Answers phone, talks on phone.

Happy, lovey kid.

Enjoys Relationships.

Affectionate

RAYMOND

Collects Key chains, enjoys yard sales.

Gross-motor activity

Able to run errands, Do chores around house

Uses Microwave, fixes drinks on own, Did things in Kitchen.

Polite to people

Sensitive to others

Perceptive

Moves Furniture

* MEDICINES HAVE LESSENED HIS ACTIVITY SCHEDULE.

R.A. 10·17·91

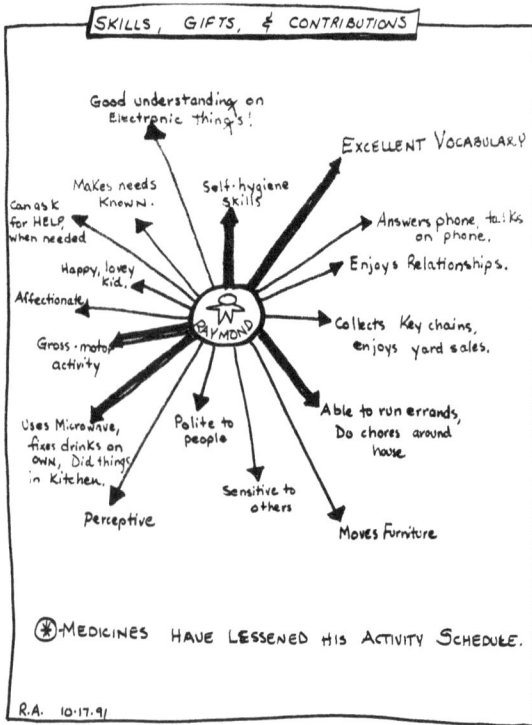

by Jo Ann and Hope in their early discussions with Betty, Raymond and Jim. They detailed Raymond's current life, his history, his network of relationships, his and his family's dreams. With this information in place, everyone at the early meetings could see what they were working with, and they could jump out of the usual and build a plan for Raymond out of the information gathered and the creative ideas of the group at each meeting.

Raymond's mother, Betty, said it best. She called it "blank paper" planning. She said she had never had the opportunity to start from scratch in identifying what Raymond needed. She'd never dared to look at his prospects in a totally new and different way.

The human service system's response had always been to go through a list of programs that were available, like group homes* or planned day programs or sheltered workshops.* Staff members would then try to explain to Betty why Raymond would not be well served in them. And they were right; he would not have been well served.

With the papers on the walls and the general agenda

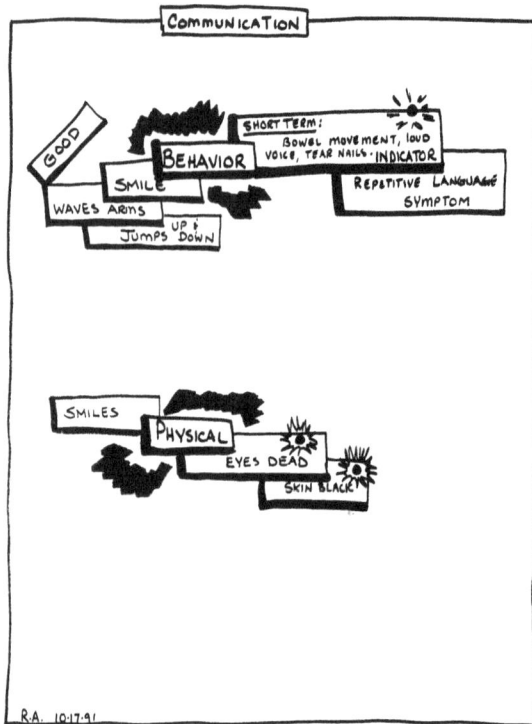

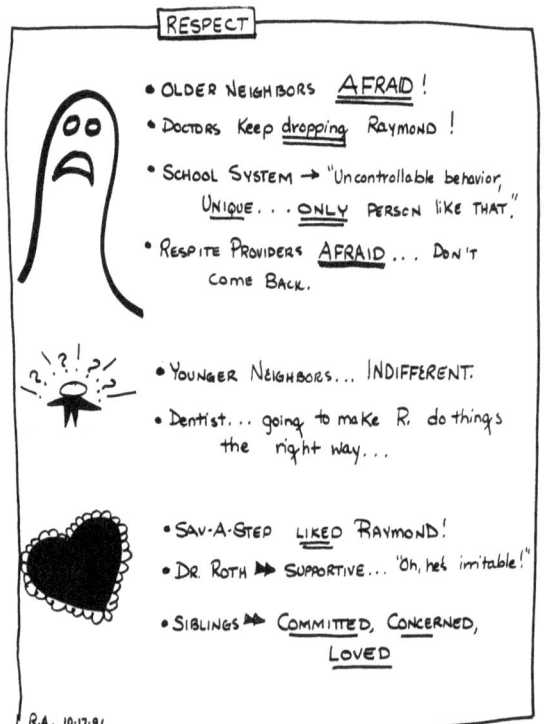

COMMUNICATION

GOOD

BEHAVIOR

SMILE

WAVES ARMS

JUMPS UP & DOWN

SHORT TERM: BOWEL MOVEMENT, LOUD VOICE, TEAR NAILS. INDICATOR

REPETITIVE LANGUAGE SYMPTOM

SMILES

PHYSICAL

EYES DEAD

SKIN BLACK

R.A. 10·17·91

RESPECT

• OLDER NEIGHBORS AFRAID!

• DOCTORS Keep dropping RAYMOND!

• SCHOOL SYSTEM → "Uncontrollable behavior, UNIQUE... ONLY PERSON like THAT."

• RESPITE PROVIDERS AFRAID... DON'T COME BACK.

• YOUNGER NEIGHBORS... INDIFFERENT.

• Dentist... going to make R. do things the right way...

• SAV-A-STEP LIKED RAYMOND!

• DR. ROTH ▶ SUPPORTIVE... "Oh, he's imitable!"

• SIBLINGS ▶ COMMITTED, CONCERNED, LOVED

R.A. 10·17·91

sketched out in pictures, the group began to open their minds to look at what could be done.

Jo Ann applied markers to paper on December 18, 1991. She opened the agenda with this item:

"Carolyn went with Raymond to Biggs and they tried out a scooter to see if Raymond would like to use one." She draws the little scooter on the sheet.

Betty added, "Tim visited Raymond. They talked a while. I think Raymond likes Tim. Chuck Skyles came to see Raymond. He asked Raymond if he wanted to go out to see Chuck's car, the first time. Raymond said no. But when Chuck came back, Raymond went out to the car. We've noticed that when a new person comes to see Raymond, he ignores them. If they'll persist, then he'll eventually warm to them."

Jo Ann drew Tim and Chuck on the paper, and gave a flourish to a little car for Chuck. Betty talked about Milton coming to visit Raymond. Milton said that he wanted to find out what things Raymond really liked. Another little person was drawn on the friendship part of the chart. That figure began to "do" new and different things as Jo Ann asked for more ideas. Ideas were played with that months before would never have been considered as possible in Raymond's life.

At a pause in the conversation Betty invited people to have more grapes or some cheese and crackers. "Anybody need anything else to drink?"

Tim reported that he spoke with Trude Scharff at Citizen Advocacy* to find an advocate for Raymond. Phil Coffen, Raymond's neighbor, served on the Advocacy committee. He would look into recruiting. A picture of the CA office went up on the paper.

Jo Ann taped another paper up as discussion opened on funding. Little dollar signs surrounded notes about the next subjects. Tim talked about an upcoming Supported Living* meeting and then explained about other newly available state funding.

Tim added, "There is a possibility that Home and Community Based Waiver* funds might be obtained through Visiting Nurses.* That could pay for seven hours a month of respite time. I want to find out if we can supply the staff and they can administer the funds."

Tim's task would be to follow up on that. Jo Ann drew a Tim figure and VNA on the task list.

Lucy Axton reported that she did some research and was right that Raymond was not appropriately funded with his SSI (Supplemental Security Income, usually state supplemented funding for people living with disabilities*). Betty had no response from SSI so Lucy got a lawyer to look into this.

The meeting continued as each member reported on the outcome of the tasks they had done. The little pictures were drawn, illustrating fresh ideas to pull Raymond into a new level of contact with other people, his neighborhood and activities that he could begin to enjoy. Betty was stunned that the "blank-paper" planning had so many ideas piling up on Raymond's behalf. She was fascinated that the pictures seemed to make the ideas more feasible and do-able.

Raymond's group did not suddenly cohere and become an effective working group. The process of bringing together a variety of people to find what would work was long and ongoing. There was often a sense of walking into a dark cave with one tiny flashlight, everyone holding hands for dear life, even for the old "hands" from human services who were pioneers in person-centered planning

This group pushed on through the cave. What, in that first tense meeting in the community center with Jo Ann, Tim, Milton, Hope, Lucy, Raymond, and the rest of Betty's family and friends, prompted ten years of connection, struggle, work, confusion, tears, excitement, innovation, and joy? A dream? A family, dreaming of a better situation for their son? Was it the unusual strength and love of a determined mother who, while she didn't always know how to make the best happen for her son, knew instinctively how to connect with people in a way that made them want to do the best for Raymond?

Even though the group focused on the positive, that focus had to be an active, creative, and persistent generation of energy toward things getting better. Without that energy, entropy and a sense of passivity could easily settle in and discourage everyone. Jo Ann Boyle got the group started with a clarity and energy that defined its direction for much of its years of gathering.

"Jo Ann had the vision," Tim Estes said. That may be what brought such a commonality to the group. We bought into her vision, and that gave it consistency. Personnel changed from year to year, and sometimes month to month, but the people who became a part of this, no matter what their personal or professional role, said, 'This is the vision we bought; this is what we want to see happen for Raymond.' When you have people who commit to that it is amazing what can happen. People who said Raymond would never do this or do that had defined his life up to that point. I don't think Betty ever believed those people."

It was necessary for this group of people to crawl together out of and over the expectations that are often set by cultural beliefs about what can happen for people with serious disabilities. In doing so, they were able to see Raymond as himself and not a bundle of diagnoses that artificially define those expectations. There was a constant need to refresh this perception because it is only too easy to fall back into the "trance" of "how it is," the collective beliefs of an apparently indifferent society. The graphic process probed new territory of thought and creativity and pushed the group into their best "heads" to think in a fresh way about what could be made to happen on Raymond's particular path.

Being committed

Even with the constantly renewed perspective, there is also the problem of holding such a group together consistently. People aren't very consistent. People move, change jobs, take on other responsibilities, and even occasionally lose heart or fall into grief. This is a persistent concern in a group like Raymond's and it requires energy to continue to pull a group back together in the face of such setbacks.

Carolyn Wheeler put it this way: "There was Jo Ann Boyle, but she moved away, and later Hope left. As other people left, I had this feeling, 'Who was ultimately going to still be here?' It was Betty Atherton. We all did make a contribution and it wouldn't have happened without that. But there is a reality here; when you distill it down, when the rubber meets the road, it would be family. Because we all could leave, and family couldn't or wouldn't."

Frankly, family or advocates who make a family-like commitment to following a person's life are the most effective support for people with developmental disabilities.

Carolyn Wheeler is a good example of one person making a family-like commitment to another. When she was working with people with disabilities for Seven Counties Services, she met a man who was living in what could best be described as dire circumstances. She became his advocate and pulled together community resources for him. She moved Clinton from "a warehouse for marginalized people" into a family home to be cared for. Over time, Carolyn oversaw most everything that happened to Clinton and welcomed him into her family as a social friend. She engineered his getting a new job in a much more congenial situation than his previous workshop employment. Even after Carolyn moved to another city, she regularly visited Clinton and continued her close monitoring of his life. She included him in family activities, making his occasions

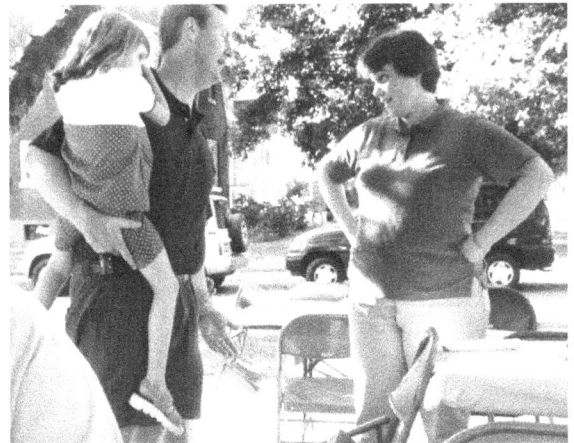

Carolyn Wheeler at a fish fry with David Block and daughter.

part of her family's celebrations. Clinton's life was lived on an entirely different plane of experience, work, social engagement, and fun because Carolyn had befriended him and become his advocate. She knew personally what hard work that could be. She wanted the same kind of support for Raymond and his family. She later became an integral part of Raymond's group. Raymond and Clinton became friends.

An advocate like Carolyn becomes like family to an adult with disabilities. And like families, these relationships are all different and each unique. But they are all marked by a commitment to a person from another person who will see that needs are met.

"I always loved John O'Brien's definition of Citizen Advocacy," says Tim, who has worked developing advocacy relationships. 'Citizen Advocacy is a way of organizing surprises.' That's a good definition of what a real person-centered* group should be."

"And this was such a creative group," Betty observes. "They managed right off to think up several ways to get Raymond out of the house. Lucy Axton took on getting sufficient SSI payments. Milton Tyree and Chuck Skyles developed ways for Raymond to make contacts out in the community. I had knots in my stomach worrying about the effect that Raymond's difficult behavior might have on the members. I dreaded that the group would just disappear. But they didn't.

"It was ever so gradual, but I became a believer in those blank pieces of paper as foundations for the creative thinking in the group. No one but us will ever know what those filled papers did for our family. I would think, 'If only Raymond would have had this type of group supporting him when he was little!'"

Chapter 3

Out REACH

Raymond and his family didn't have support when he was little. When Raymond was born, children born with disabilities often were not identified early enough for appropriate intervention. Even now parents are usually too busy with basic survival issues to research and contact necessary supports, assuming that such supports exist.

While people who live and work with children with developmental disabilities know that early intervention can be totally life-changing for a child, the community as a whole may not recognize this. There is a two-sided cultural message that many parents encounter about their children with disabilities. One side subtly negates the family for having a disabled child; the other side of the message taps into the "special" poster child pity-evoking, charity provoking image of children with disabilities. Neither of these attitudes in any way encourages a family to build a life enriched with the best that can be offered for their child.

In the U.S., public programs such as Head Start and First Steps, which offer solid early support for children, have been losing funding. Parents who have found such programs helpful for their children are distraught that these services have been targeted for deep cuts. Early and intense stimulation and awareness training can mean the difference between a child being able to benefit from school, or being "warehoused" in poor quality classrooms for an entire school career.

Such programs were not even available for Raymond, and his school experiences were largely negative and a strain on him and his family. Private programs such as REACH were not around when Raymond was small, but through Jo Ann Boyle and Hope Dittmeier he was able to benefit as a young adult from their unique approach to making things work for young people with disabilities.

Hope wanted Betty to know right away that "REACH wasn't a service provider. We were facilitating and coordinating. We didn't have the intention or the ability to serve Raymond. We were funded to go out into the state and launch efforts that would pull people into this particular planning process. So it wasn't like an agency initiating a service, like providing day programming or a residential placement. It was a unique project. The model for the Outreach program was not that Raymond was the client.

The client of that project was the support network around him. It was very clear that we weren't about to change Raymond, or give prescribed clinical service to Raymond. It was a service to the network of people who wanted to support him."

There could be a fit here for Raymond and his family who were already a strong support circle for him. Raymond could benefit from Hope's expertise and Jo Ann's facilitation. Raymond and his family could set the course for whatever support or assistance would be offered by recruited outsiders. Despite Betty's best efforts up to this time, she hadn't been able to get stable support from any local programs. Perhaps that was a disguised blessing; often programs try to fit people into their mold rather than developing a program to fit the person. And the latter model would definitely be Betty's preference.

As Hope Dittmeier from REACH said, "The vision for Raymond took a long time to get to and took a long time to work on. I remember originally we'd have fewer dark days and his world would be a little bit bigger. But we didn't know anything more than that. I think a lot of the process of figuring that out helped build this group. So often you go in and people are pretty clear. They know what they want. Then you go to the work of making it happen.

"But this group had to spend a lot of time trying to figure out what were the possibilities. They got to know Raymond slowly. It took many years to get to the idea of 'What would a good day look like for Raymond?' It didn't come easy; it took a lot of time."

Looking at the ideas that were the foundation for REACH, we can see how Hope and Jo Ann moved Raymond's group in a direction that would focus on Raymond's priorities, and not the agendas of serving agencies.

This statement from REACH reflects what the family and his group sees as ideal, but possible goals. These ideals form a framework out of which they can develop services that suit Raymond where he is, and that can be modified as his world grows and changes:

> Services are available in close proximity and are accessible without reference to physical, psychological, social, linguistic, or other barriers; services are comprehensive and appropriate, in that they possess features that address priority needs the family has identified, at a level of service sufficient to their need; services are formulated and delivered at a high level of quality such that the family perceives them as an organized whole and can participate in a consistent and effective manner; services serve to promote psychological competence and self-sufficiency rather than focusing exclusively on dysfunction and pathology.

The group worked in the context of Raymond's neighborhood and family to provide what he needed, and they gradually decided and juggled and networked to bring in the people and services he would need to make the best of what he wanted in life. Raymond's involvement in his local community was emphasized. Several of his circle members lived close by. Many of his daily activities took place in businesses and other locations in his neighborhood.

From the very beginning of the group's organizing around Raymond, the emphasis was on Raymond's participation in decisions. Everyone focused on listening to his needs and desires, even if that involved some extremely subtle communication. There was always a need to balance what Raymond was trying to express with what his family needed, and what the group and family's goals were for Raymond. This is person-centered planning, with extraordinary family support. The group would constantly reach for effective social integration for Raymond, and spend time finding ways to help Raymond manage his behavior to make his contacts with his social world less of a problem.

While this would appear in the context of services for people with disabilities to be an innovative approach to planning one's days, and one's life, is it any different from the way we best work with our typical family members to support them in their life decisions? Why do we think planning for people with disabilities is so different from planning for most everyone else?

Chapter 4

Reach Out

The hotel was tall and the central atrium rose from the ground all the way to the skylight at the top. It was airy, bright with filtered winter sun, and hung all around with sun-soaking plants in pots. This one afternoon the plants seemed to quiver just a bit as the atrium echoed with "BACK OFF," and BUG OUT," and other similar and stronger expressions rolling up and down like thunder from the eighth floor.

Raymond was visiting Atlanta with Betty, Hope, Hope's sister-in-law Ann, and Jim Schrecker, his day program coordinator. Hope, Ann and, tentatively, Raymond were to present at the TASH* conference. Everyone had felt that Raymond had come so far in his connecting to the community that he could come to share that success with the conference. Hope and Ann were to speak about a neighborhood walking club that Hope and others in the neighborhood had started. Ann had joined the walkers, and Betty and Raymond were also involved.

Betty described the trip with some laughs and some sighs.

"When we got to the airport Raymond grouched at Ann and I thought, 'Well, he is nervous.'

"I wouldn't go without Jim Schrecker because I was thinking I would need support for Raymond, and I was right. We got on the plane and as soon as it took off he started hollering out. Jim Schrecker is just laid back. You could light a fire under his chair and he wouldn't move. He just ignored the yelling. I was just wired to the hilt. Hope tried not to notice the hollering, but you could tell the strain on her face. The airline people seemed to take it in stride. The plane was close to being full. When we got to Atlanta I thought when we got off the plane he would stop, but it didn't stop, so we didn't ride the tram. We walked to the terminal. Raymond kept screaming and screaming. He just kept hollering; I don't know how he kept his voice. I thought it would be better to take a limo. But he still kept hollering. When we got to the hotel with the big atrium, Raymond's yells echoed and echoed.

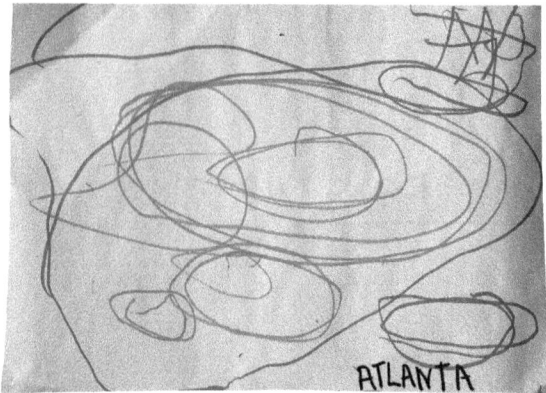

Raymond's painting "Atlanta."

"Hope said, 'Let's just go on and eat and maybe that will settle him.'

"But in the dining room he kept on hollering. Ann acted more adult and said, 'Poor Raymond, it is a shame.' We were really proud of her. I heard later that Hope feared we would get locked up. She probably called Carolyn Wheeler a dozen times while we were there. She talked to John O'Brien. He said he would like to see Raymond.

"Raymond didn't sleep well that night. He kept having to go to the bathroom and woke me up each time. Jim Schrecker wanted to know if he could have the next afternoon off; then after that he would be there for Raymond. So Raymond and I stayed in the room and he just was very nattery. But the next morning he was hollering out at the breakfast table again. We had a wonderful waitress who talked directly to Raymond and that toned him down a little bit.

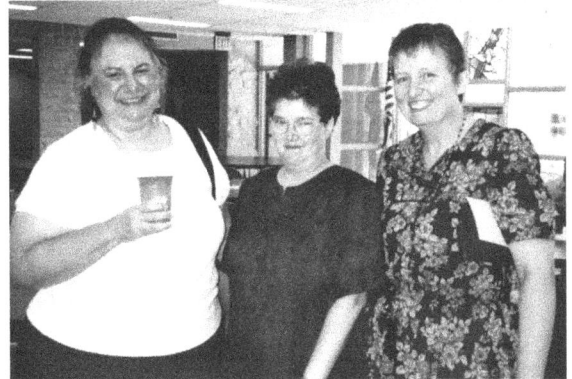

Nancy Brucchieri, Ann Dittmeier, and Julie Cole.

"After breakfast we ran into John O'Brien and he kept looking at Raymond. He talked a little bit to him, but he never took his eyes off of him. I don't know what that was about. You could tell by the look on Raymond's face, things weren't good.

"That evening Jim stayed with Raymond, and Hope and I went to the Mall to make things a little lighter. I knew Jim was getting frustrated when we got back. He said, 'Let's get a van and drive back.'

"I said, 'No, an hour on the plane is better than ten in the van.'

"By coincidence my niece Linda from California was presenting about nursing at another conference in Atlanta. She kept calling Jim's room thinking it was my room. Jim and I had switched rooms so that Raymond had the quieter room. Linda finally got through to us and I told her that things were tough. She came right over to support us. There were a few bright spots.

"I thought when we headed home things would be better. While I had a smoke, my tranquilizer, before we got on the plane, Jim asked the attendants if we could board first onto the economy flight. They had heard Raymond and said, 'OK, fine.'

"They gave us the first seat so we could get off first. But Raymond started hollering as soon as the plane took off. The attendants would bring a bag of peanuts and he would eat them quietly, and then holler out, again.

"When we got back into Louisville it was a rainy, wet day and I couldn't remember where I had put my car in the parking lot. I told Raymond he was just going to have to be patient till I was able to find the car. He was so glad to be back that he was a trooper about finding the car.

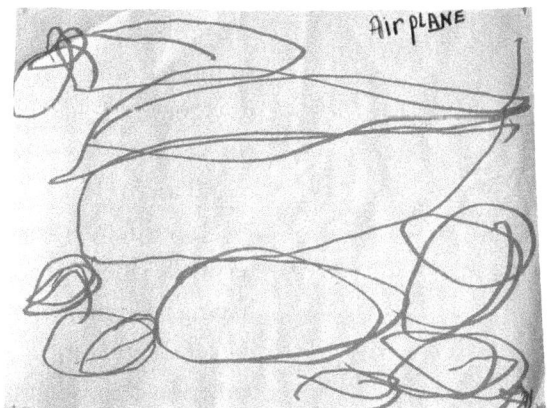

Raymond's painting "Airplane."

"When we got home he said, 'I've got to call Milton.'

"'I'm home,' he told Milton, and then he said he had to call Nancy. He wanted to make sure that they were still friends. But he didn't tell them anything he'd done. He told them he had a good time."

In a Supported Living Grant request proposal, Betty would later describe the trip like this: "For three days Raymond continuously (really) expressed himself in a boisterous manner using vulgar language and generally creating a turbulent time for all. After returning to Louisville Raymond had heightened anxiety. He worried intensely about many small things like whether his air conditioner would be reinstalled. He worried about that from December to June. 'Are you going to be here in June?' he would ask continuously.

"I think the good that came out of that time was that when we got back Hope called Herb Lovett, the renowned Boston psychologist who worked primarily with people with complicated developmental disabilities. He said he was going to be in town, or in Cincinnati, soon and would meet with us. It was good to have the connection with Herb Lovett.

"I was surprised at Raymond's reaction to the trip because when we went to California on a plane he was fine. He enjoyed the plane ride. I don't know why it was different; maybe because then he was going to see Carolyn and Gerald. But when we were coming back from a layover in Atlanta on the California trip, the weather was really rough and stormy, very bumpy, and Raymond was going 'Whee, whee!' with delight when we'd hit the bumps. Denise and I laughed, because everybody else was turning green at the gills. He was in his late teens then. That's why I was really surprised. But on the way back from TASH he did say on the plane, 'Don't fall out of the sky.'"

"I think about the trip to Atlanta a lot," said Hope. "You know if you don't go to the pediatrician's office with your children bumped and bruised now and again, you are probably overprotecting them. I think there were some times that things didn't so go well with Raymond. The trip wasn't necessarily a terrible thing to have done. Raymond's life had been so small. While helping him have a bigger world, if we didn't run into problems we were probably being overprotective. I don't think taking Raymond to TASH was a mistake."

"It was harder than we thought it was going to be." Carolyn Wheeler added. "Afterwards when we got back, he would talk about going; I think he was proud about having been invited. Some of the time he had a good time. I think it made his world bigger. There were tough moments. But I don't think it was the wrong thing to do. The same way that we didn't know when it was not safe, none of us knew where that line was until we got close enough to it to say, 'Oops!'

"Raymond always had people around him when things got difficult, people around him who loved him, cared about him and wanted to do those things they could to support him," Carolyn continued. "And there's not much more you can ask for any of us. I've stepped beyond what I believed I am capable of doing at times, and it's been good to have people around me to help. Raymond's hard times were so dramatic. But it's really no different than anyone else's life. There are times one goes over the edge.

"If we had created a life for Raymond where he hadn't any anxiety, he would have been at home all the time. That would have been the worse thing to have done."

"We convinced Raymond to do all kinds of things," Milton added. "Like going to TASH. 'C'mon Raymond, it'll be great!' After Raymond had called me and told me how marvelously it had gone. I said, 'I knew it would go well.' And everybody's face went, UNNNNN!?!! But Raymond said, when I asked how it went. 'Great!'"

"Betty, he was glad he went." Hope agreed.

Aunt Mary's Visit

Aunt Mary is coming in on a plane.
Raymond is going to take the car to the airport.
Mother is going to drive.
Mother has to have the key to the car.
Mother will start the car.
She will open the garage door with the button.
The garage light goes on.
And then the garage door opens.
Mother then takes the car out.
We go to pick up Meemaw.
Gerald and Sandy are coming.
It is Friday and we will get Mary at the airport.
I am not going to shout at the airport.
I will feel fine at the airport.
I will be a gentleman and I will have fun.
Mary will come from the plane.
She will have a suitcase and luggage and a bag.
She will pack her suitcase.
She will get in the car with Meemaw, Raymond, and Mother.
We will drive to our house.

Chapter 5

Choices?

I t is a long drive out to the far suburbs and the two women are unusually quiet during the entire trip. Mother and daughter, they are going together for mutual support to consider an option which neither is comfortable about. But people have told them this may be the only option they have. When they park the car in the small lot and walk up to the large doors of the big rambling building, they look at each other and sigh.

A man meets them in the lobby-like area and asks their names and smiles at them. He says he will show them around the residences, if they would like that. They walk down a long hall and he shows them rooms where people are gathered at tables and focused on craft activities, or simply sitting and watching as the visitors look around.

"That's where they have arts and crafts. Most of them just sit and ignore what's going on. But that's how it is. Now I'll show you the gym."

The ladies are led into a big cinderblock room with a linoleum floor. Basketball hoops hang from backboards suspended from the ceiling and the tiled floor is at least marked appropriately. There are mats piled up on the side. But no one is using the room. Dana drags her foot on the linoleum and looks skeptically at her mother.

"They have ball games here and once a month the staff organizes a dance for them. They seem to like that. Anyway."

Down the windowed corridor they head toward a large central room that is flanked by halls of rooms radiating out. No one is anywhere to be seen.

"This is one of the halls. There are five with eight rooms around them. Some of the rooms are double, but most are single. There are plans in the future for apartments to be built where two to four people will live. They will be very nice. But that is down the road. I think Mary Smith might be home. I'll show you her space."

They go down a short dim hall and into a little room. A woman sits in a wheelchair looking at a small television. Her room is clean and cluttered with a chintz spread on the little hospital-style bed and matching curtains that seem to fill the space with color. There is a crowd of dolls and stuffed animals on her small dresser top. Mary doesn't seem to notice the intrusion at first, but then looks up at the visitors and smiles.

"Hi. This is my room. That's my bed, my dresser. Those are my dolls. That's my TV."

"Well, thank you for showing us your things. And your name is Mary?"

"Yes'm. And this is my room."

"Well, Mary, do you like living here?"

"Yes'm"

"What do you like to do on your own time?"

Betty suspects that Mary might have a great deal of her own time. Mary looks at Betty and Dana and back at her TV. The young man briskly ushers them out the door and down the hall. Most of the doors are closed, so they don't look into the other rooms.

"They don't have a lot to say. But don't you think the room is nice? This is the bathroom for this hall." They are quickly ducked into a large terrazzo floored room with open showers all along one wall, and urged right out before they get a good look.

"What kind of schedule do the residents keep? There don't seem to be many people here today."

"Most of them work at the sheltered workshop. And you saw some at the craft room. They keep them busy."

"Doing what?" Dana sincerely wanted to know, but looked askance at Betty as the young man leads them down another long hall.

"Oh, this and that. They do little crafts and if those turn out nice they sell them at little sales, or in the front hall area. The workshops that most residents work at are separate locations. Are you thinking of placing your child here? Some of these kids have been here since we opened and are just as happy as they can be."

"Well, we are just looking around today."

After a quick look at the dining area, Betty and Dana give each other the eye sign and begin to take their leave of the tour guide. He shows them down the hall and back to the front doors.

"If you want any other information, or another chance to look around, just give us a call. I am sorry our director wasn't here today to talk to you. He is at a week-long conference out of town. Here is my card. I look forward to talking with you again."

"I don't." Betty mutters as she and Dana made a bee-line for the car.

"I don't know about you, but I had a bad feeling about that place," Betty tells Dana as she backs the car out of the lot and back onto the road.

"Well, it was clean and all and the few people we saw seemed healthy, but everybody looked bored and gloomy. Even the lady whose job it seems to be to show off her room seemed bored, and disconnected. I didn't see any kids. What was that about 'your child,' and 'these kids'?"

"Did you notice that the man never referred to the residents as friends or associates. It was always they and them. That gave me a real bad feeling."

Betty didn't go back, even though several people had told her that the residence she visited was one of the nicest in the area and so many people were pleased that their children had been able to move there.

A Conversation In the Group About Choices

Many years after that visit Betty told the group during a meeting, "As Raymond was growing up we had a tremendous lot of hope that we could make his life useful for him or something that would be successful for him. But as he got older his behavior got so bizarre. They told us to go see that facility. So Dana and I went out to see it, when Raymond was around 17.

"But Raymond was one of us. When that man went around with us at the institution and talked to the people the way he did, we thought, 'They need to get rid of him; he has no respect or use for any of the people there.' We felt like institutions were scary. Then when things got more bizarre for Raymond, we said, 'What are we going to do?'"

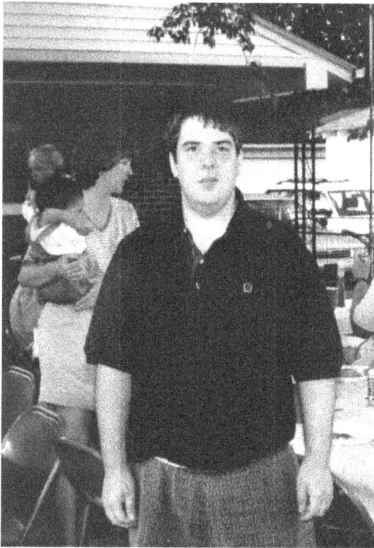

Behind Raymond is Hope Dittmeier with daughter Nikki.

"I remember one of the things that kept me going," Hope said about those times when things didn't seem to be working for Raymond even when his family and his circle were doing their best to pull for him.

"I remember a scene in the movie *Awakenings,* about the neurologist/author Dr. Oliver Sacks, played by Robin Williams. There is a very distinct scene in that movie where these doctors and others are criticizing Dr. Sacks for administering medication which temporarily reanimated his patients. 'Well, what are you doing? What were you thinking when you gave these people hope?' And the camera zooms in and he looks over his shoulder; it's very dramatic, and he says, 'Because the alternative is unthinkable.' I remember I just kept thinking we must keep going, we don't have any choice here, the alternative isn't OK. So you sit back at the table and you keep doing it any way whether it is working or not, because the alternative was not ever, ever a possibility."

Cindy Bayes became a member of Raymond's group when Raymond was being served through Supports for Community Living (funding from the Medicaid Waiver for people at risk of institutionalization.*), administered by Seven Counties Services. As program manager, she assigned support coordinators to Raymond's group and became more involved as she watched the creative methods that the group used to make the Supports money work the way Raymond needed it to work. As a member of the support group, Cindy was aware that Raymond's family had made a clear choice that living in the community would work for him, no matter how much effort it took on their part to make that happen. As a person with a family member living with serious disability, Cindy had deep experience of making choices like those Betty had been facing.

Betty's talk about the Athertons' choice against Raymond moving to an institution got Cindy to reminiscing. "We believed our disabled sister should live in the community too," she said, "but it was because we had a lot of natural support. As much as we believed and trusted our pediatrician who made home visits to her, and didn't make house calls to others, there did come a time that he recommended we look at a facility.

"'You don't have a wheelchair; you're carrying her around; she's twelve; she is getting heavy. You need to go and at least look at some things.'

"Nobody wanted that, but we did go to look. It was so heart-sickening to see those places. They were deplorable. After one visit, we all went out in the car and nobody said anything. We sat out in the car crying. And we went home, we got a new bedroom suite, new this, new that, we were digging in. That is why we wanted to make life at home for our sister work.

"So Betty, why did your family want community life for Raymond instead of a facility," Cindy asked. "What influences were helping you all to see that? How did that become your mind-set, the set of glasses you were seeing through?"

"You all were life-savers when Jo Ann came in," Betty answered.

"We wanted to have an alternative. We knew, as nice as everyone said that facility was, we were not comfortable with the place. I think most people would want the best for their family member. We didn't see that being the best for Raymond.

"Raymond wanted to be someplace where he was needed and he wouldn't have been needed at a residential facility," Milton said, supporting Betty's idea.

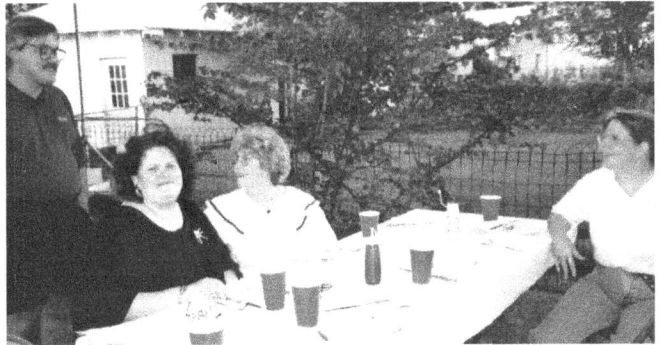

From left, Gerry Stribling, Linda Mc-Cauliffe, Cindy Bayes, and Dana Atherton Labhart.

Carolyn Wheeler continued, "He would not have stayed there. This is just an opinion. But when people have significant behavior problems, if their behaviors do not improve after treatment, they are gone. That private facility doesn't provide lifetime security. In public institutions, nobody can kick you out, like at Hazelwood or Oakwood. [Unless, of course, the state moves to close down those institutions due to allegations of abuse, or to loss of funding by Medicaid. And this became a serious issue in Kentucky in 2006.]

"It is interesting to hear you talk about this, Betty." Carolyn continued.

"I guarantee you we could have this conversation about living in institutions vs. living out in the community with other parents, and they would feel the opposite extreme. They believe that the community is scary and the institution is wonderful and is safe and secure and 'My family member is so well treated and has been happy there for thirty years.' So where is the truth? People can have the exact same experience and radically different perspectives about the exact same thing and both feel it so deeply."

"Carolyn, don't you think they didn't want to see what we saw? They only saw what they wanted to see?" Betty wondered.

The Key: What Works For People

One set of family members goes to a residential facility or a nursing home and sees a kind of care that they feel will support their family member in a way that they can be pleased with or at least tolerate. Some families insist that their disabled family member be kept in an institution. They deeply fear what would happen to their disabled relatives if they had to live out in the community. How would they be adequately cared for? Who would be in charge of their physical needs? Don't they need special kinds of therapy and treatment that they could only get in a facility?

Another family goes to see such a facility and sees a lack of life, a boring existence, inadequate care and nourishment and people starving for attention and interest in their lives. They deeply fear what would happen to their relative if they had to live in the facility.

Hope says, "This is a values decision, and people just have different views."

Hope's sister-in-law, Ann, lives not far from Betty's home. Her family helped her buy a nice little duplex in a comfortable neighborhood. A family lives in the downstairs apartment. She spends time with them and they look after the house and check on her and often share meals with her. She is busy in the community, working for pay several days a week in a department store, volunteering in a nearby nursing facility for elderly religious women, and ushering at the Center for the Arts. She walks and takes the city buses where she needs to go, and is visited regularly by her support coordinator. They love to do each other's nails and have dinner out and do volunteer jobs together. At home she enjoys reading, artwork, and making rosaries. She spends a lot of time visiting her large family. Her situation was one of the models for the group as they explored ideas with Raymond and his family about his goals. She lives as anyone would in her neighborhood. The difference is that several people, paid and unpaid, stay a little closer to her as she moves through her week, and her family supports her as they would any family member, but with more oversight.

Perhaps Hope's perspective and values were deeply influenced by what she experienced first-hand in her first job.

"I was 17 years old and went to work in an institution, and I knew some things there were horribly wrong," Hope remembers. "I didn't have the words for it. I was just a kid in my first job, and I looked around. I was freaking out, 'There is a problem here!'

"I quit and went home. I couldn't stay there under those conditions. It wasn't just a decision. It was an emotional reaction. 'This is not right!'

"It had nothing to do with labels. I just knew you don't line naked people up and give them baths in rows down the hallway. Something was not right about that. But other people worked there and thought things like that were fine. I couldn't figure that out.

"I think it is true – whether you are talking about family members of people with disability, or people who work in the field – that we need to have a sense that this work is about justice and civil rights for *anyone.* This goes beyond the issue of disability."

Putting your family member in an institutional setting or finding an appropriate home for her in the community is historically a choice that has set family members against each other, community services at "war," and people with different ideological stances on opposite firing lines.

Carolyn talks about ideology and perception. She says that two groups of people can see the same circumstances laid out before them and react in totally different ways.

"You can have the same information, but a very different reality. This has to do with your fundamental values and beliefs. What you see about services or programs or institutions for your disabled family member gets filtered through your set of fundamental beliefs and values.

"There is a shifting that can occur, and does occur for families, like some of those hundred families currently newly involved in the Supports for Community Living Waiver, who had family members in institutions. They have since left the institutions. Many of those families have become the strongest advocates for community services. The change in their attitudes was not an event; it was a shifting over time as things worked for the people they cared about. Perhaps that is the key; what really works for people.

"Because what works is what people will want for the protection of their family member and for the enhancement of their lives."

"There was a huge difference between what you all did, Betty," Carolyn continues, "and what happens for the families whose family members choose institutions. I think the difference is the level of involvement. And it is a vast difference. For a family whose relative lives in an institution, the institution does do it all. When staff don't show up there won't be a phone call. When physical or behavioral problems occur, you are not awakened in the middle of the night with an emergency. Betty, think of all the calls that you had and all the things that you had to respond to and all the doctors' appointments you arranged, or were frustrated at not getting. You had daily involvement, even hourly involvement, and that would not have been the case if Raymond had been in an institution."

"I think there is an REM song," says Hope, "that says not everyone can carry the weight of the world, and I do think there are a lot of families that simply couldn't do this. And to make something like this happen takes even more extraordinary effort and energy and resources than just the day-to-day care. Not everybody can do it. Not everybody can or wants to. Not everybody has the skills.

"I used the terms 'being open' and 'flexible,' but the bottom line is, Betty, you were very sophisticated in managing to invite all these people into your lives. You warmly embraced us and questioned us. And you were cautious when you thought we were nuts, but you handled that beautifully. You could have just as easily kept people from coming back. What you did to welcome this group in is a fairly sophisticated thing to make happen and there are a lot of families that don't have the desire or the sophistication to do it."

Hope continues, "What we are describing here could help a lot of families that have the resources to do what Raymond's family did. But there will be a lot of families that can't choose that route. Frankly, folks who have had the life experience that Raymond had might daunt agencies that would try to deal with their needs. I am not confident that many agencies or human service organizations would be able to deal with the level of complication that a situation like Raymond's would require. The only times I have seen success like Raymond's was when family was intensively involved."

"I wanted to share this point as we were talking about values-based attitudes and perceptions," says Cindy Bayes.

"If at some point in the group's support of Raymond, Betty was exhausted, as she often was, and the family was at wit's end and no one knew what to do, someone in the group might have suggested, 'Let's just put Raymond in a facility for a couple of weeks of respite.' And then the family rests, recovers and gets their senses back. You know that at that point it would be a lot easier for him to stay there in the facility. 'I kind of like it around here when somebody's able to sleep all night.'

"It could have been very seductive. All of us in the group had to have a strong sense about keeping Raymond in his home, in the community. None of us could let down our guard and say, 'Let's put him in respite.' It helps me to see how vulnerable the family is to listening to anything when they are exhausted and out of ideas and everybody who comes to help is exhausted and out of ideas. You just might listen to anybody."

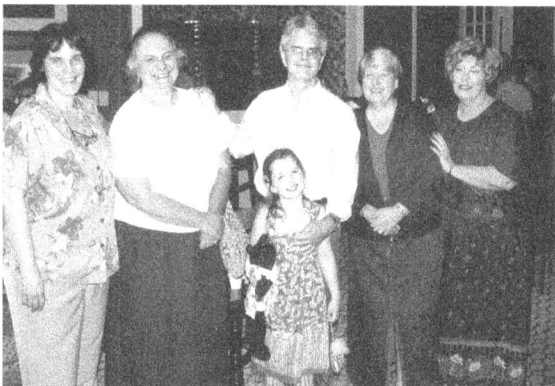

From left, Carolyn Wheeler, Nancy Bruscchieri, Milton and Kaylyn Tyree, Darcy Elks, and Cindy Bayes.

"But we, the whole family, couldn't have known what the options could be," says Betty.

"I remember saying to Jim that the group had other ideas, different ideas. That was interesting. I said to Jim, 'I can't imagine what they have in mind.'

"But I am not creative, and I couldn't imagine. Then when I would see a change in Raymond's life, I was happy. Then I could start seeing past that. At the beginning I just thought it was interesting, because I couldn't imagine how it would be. As it went on, it was wonderful."

The group members wondered what Betty meant when she said she was not imaginative. The whole family is creative and imaginative, and welcoming. They put a lot of energy and creativity into making things fun for each other, and making them work for Raymond.

Can any family do what Raymond's family did to make his life what he and they most wanted for him? The group believed that with the right supports and enough energy this could be done, but the key is what works for the person and for the people supporting that person.

I Moved Furniture   February 28, 1996

I am happy.
I moved furniture.
I cried,
No, I didn't cry.
I am happy
I am happy about me.
My TV is in my room.
How's my bedroom doing?
My TV table. I knocked it off. I knocked it onto the floor.
It didn't break, I plugged it in.
My mouth was sad. So I cried.
Do you cry Nancy?
Sometimes I cry.
I am happy.
I am going to be lucky.
Because I am happy.
I slammed the door.
Then I shut it easy.
I didn't want to get on Daddy's nerves.
Daddy would appreciate that.
I didn't beat on the light switch today.
I fixed it.
I fixed it fine.
It did not break.

Chapter 6

Family Matters

That's a wedding I'll never forget. It was different." The mother of the bride laughs and remembers that proud day when her beautiful elfin daughter with the wreathed curly hair and warm smile walked down the tiny aisle of the gaudy Tahoe chapel to meet her groom. Charming in a tea-length Victorian dress, and clutching a slightly wilted bouquet of white and salmon roses, Carolyn joined Syd under the plush red velvet canopy. Her aunt Mary beamed and her dad, Jim, smiled as the vows were exchanged. Just as the minister, Rev. Love, asked Carolyn "Do you take . . ." and she answered "I do!" one of the groomsmen yelled out in a rafter shattering blast, "BULLSHIT!!"

If there were any impediment to this marriage that "one should speak about now, or forever hold his peace," Raymond wanted it known that he wasn't holding his peace. Like most people who live with the tremendous anxiety and resulting behaviors that are sometimes described as autistic, Raymond was terribly uncomfortable with anything that constituted major change in his life. He probably felt he was losing his beloved sister to her Syd.

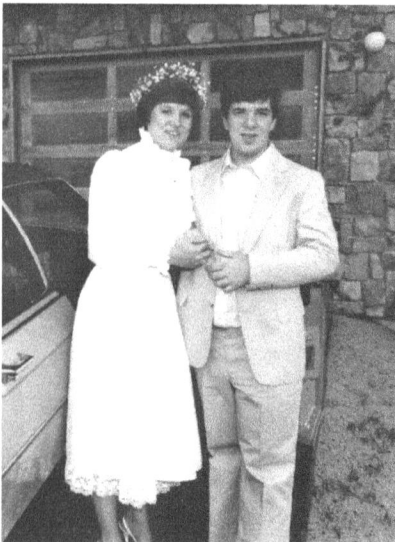

Carolyn and Raymond at her wedding.

"Well, I slept with him on my wedding night." Carolyn remembers wistfully.

"No! In Raymond's room. Seriously! Not with Syd."

Betty adds, "The next morning I said, 'Syd do you know how to play blackjack?' He said no, so I said, 'Let's go to the casino and I'll teach you.' So I took him and we sat there playing blackjack the whole damn day. They had to call us and tell us to come to supper. We were winning, the money kept coming in, until Syd got up and broke our streak."

Betty knew that it was in everyone's best interest for Carolyn to spend that day with Raymond – even if it was the day after she married Syd – so Raymond could see that she was not going away, that she would still be his sister. It had been hard enough for him to travel all the way to Tahoe.

Betty tells more of the story – a story about a family with a sense of humor and fun:

"Syd's mother had wanted them to come here and have a big wedding. Carolyn and Syd were living in California near her Aunt Mary, and she wanted her to be there. Her

Uncle Vern was having some problems with early Alzheimer's and wouldn't travel far, so they decided to have it at Tahoe.

"Syd's mother came over to our place and said, 'You all aren't going, are you?' We said, 'No, probably not.' But then Carolyn called me and said, 'We don't want to do this unless you all come and stay.' So we did. She told Raymond, 'If you wear a suit, Raymond, I'd love for you to come to my wedding.' He was anxious, though handsome in his white suit. He was thrilled to see Carolyn, but not about the marriage.

"We laughed all the way out to Tahoe about a possible big shock when we arrived.

"I had rented a house sight unseen. And my mother said, 'You don't know what you are getting.' When we got there it had two floors; a lower level with three big bedrooms and up the steps was a humongous living room area with two long, plush leather sofas and lots of chairs. It looked kind of rustic with a wooden-beamed high ceiling and big windows with a lake view. There was a little kitchen with a big counter to eat at, and a dining area, too. On that floor was a great big huge bedroom; you could have put four or five double beds in it. There was a jacuzzi and a huge walk-in closet we made a bedroom out of. Chuck slept in there because he snored so loud.

"Carolyn got married on July 2nd. We had arrived there on June 30th. When we got there and saw how big the place was we said, 'We don't need anything that big.'

"But after the wedding it turned cold, the coldest July 4th on record in Tahoe; all of the kids came to stay with us. I'd say there had to be ten boys staying with us and at times the place looked like a battlefield. That's ten plus all the rest of the family, a total of about twenty-five.

"We had sleeping bags everywhere. My mother was cooking a lot of the meals, but she didn't fix breakfast. When all those boys got up and fixed their breakfasts it was wild.

"You couldn't have planned a wedding that was any more fun than that. Kids driving into the area looking for the wedding put signs on their cars, 'If you know where Carolyn and Syd are, blow your horn,' and 'Louisville, KY to Tahoe.'

"The wedding cake was terrible. It looked like a nice two-tiered white cake with traditional bride and groom on top. Something was wrong with it. Jim took it back, but the

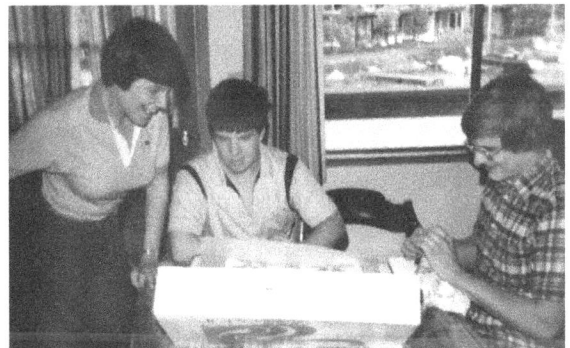

Raymond helps Carolyn and Syd open wedding presents.

people said he couldn't get a refund. So he said, 'I'll just go out and serve a piece to everyone who comes by. That will help your reputation.' They gave him his money back. The flowers were all half-dead-looking too. The baby's breath wreath for Carolyn's hair looked bedraggled. But we didn't care.

"You are probably wondering how Carolyn and Syd got to California. They were dating as they finished school at UK, but getting along ferociously, always at each other, and that was driving me crazy. I said, 'Carolyn, I can't stand this anymore. I am buying you a ticket and calling Aunt Mary and telling her you're coming out to California. You can cash the other end in or you have got a ticket to come home. You go out there and get separate from this.'

"She did go and got a job she liked. She came back to visit at Christmas time. In fact she came back twice within that year. When she went out there, Raymond got two pairs of her shoes and put them under his bed, and he put one of her purses on his bed. He missed her so. But she stayed in contact with him.

"And it like to killed Syd that she was gone. So the next February somebody said, 'You know I think Syd is thinking about going to California. Something's up.'

"So Syd rented a big truck, put his stuff in, and got Gerald to help him drive out there. Gerald stayed, too – for ten years. They said it was good. They miss California in ways."

Carolyn was never far from Raymond in her heart. She was always there for him and for her parents, even as she started her own family of little girls, Mari Elizabeth, Kelly, Traci and Sydney.

"On the way back from the wedding, Raymond really struggled to hold himself together. We stopped in Nebraska to visit our daughter Donna. By Missouri Raymond was really becoming unraveled. I was hoping to stop to visit a friend there but Raymond said over and over to his dad, 'Keep driving, Daddy; keep driving!'"

Family connections

The steamy summer night is relieved by a faint breeze over the lake. The two women are escaping in a small rowboat. One tall, slim, pretty woman with dark curly hair rows vigorously across the lake. If you were in a canoe coming up from behind their boat in the mists rising from the waters, you might be startled as you paddle past. It would seem that the same woman appears to be in the other end of the boat with a fish wriggling under her feet. The strange illusion could confuse you as you paddle toward your campsite with a story of dark night tricks of the imagination.

"I'm not taking that thing off of the hook. But it is a nice big bass!"

"Jim will do it for us. I just can't believe we got it so fast. It will taste good."

The twin sisters clamber up the bank with the still-hooked fish.

"You two! I can't believe you can't get the fish off the hook!"

"Jim, just take it off! We're going back out. It is so cool and quiet on the lake."

The campers parked on the hill above the bank are full of vacationing children, mostly sleeping or telling each other stories of the day's adventures before they nod off. The women leave their first catch and head back out on the lake. They hardly put their lines back into the water when one of the twin sisters calls out.

"You're not going to believe this. I think I've got another bite!"

They laugh and focus on playing the line to bring in the fish. Once it is in the boat,

Betty puts her foot on the jumping fish and Mary rows the boat back across the lake to the campsite.

"Oh, come on. You girls need to figure out how to get a fish off of a line if you are going out to fish after my bedtime!"

Mary and Betty both laugh at Jim, who will stay up till all hours to fish, or get up before anyone in the world, just to get the early feeders before dawn.

"Don't worry. This is too much like work. We are heading for bed."

The next evening Jim and Betty, with Denise helping, are frying up fillets of fish for all of the family and the kids' friends who are camping with them. The cornmeal smell of hot fish combines with the pine needle tang in the air, enticing youngsters to drift back to camp.

"Mom, guess what? We were trying to show Raymond how much fun the water is. Carolyn was throwing passes with the football on the beach. We were all going out to catch them, and Raymond was trying to catch a few. He backed into the water by mistake."

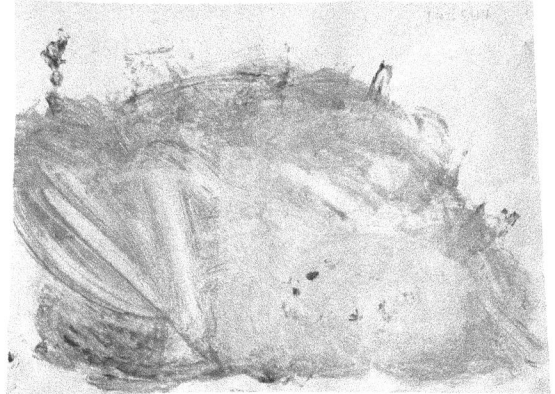

Raymond's painting "The Sun."

"Yeah, at first he got scared and screamed. But we jumped in around him and sat down in the water and eventually he sat on the edge with us. He almost liked it." Carolyn grinned her impish smile and nudged Raymond toward the picnic table full of food.

"Let's eat, Raymond."

The kids are filling plates with beans, fish, potato salad and lettuce.

Betty sits by the lake. She and Julie had driven a half hour over winding Indiana roads to be out in the brightly colored forest. It is a brisk, sunny but chilly autumn day. Betty talks about those summers in the sun with all of her children and their friends. She walks out onto a fishing pier and the wind blows her words over the lake.

"Jim started coming up here to Deam's Lake before it got developed. And he got to know the rangers. We started camping up here before they were charging anything. The rangers were great. When they started charging a fee, they would save us the campsite down the far end of the lane. We'd park there. Raymond loved the rangers' trucks. He would walk around them and examine them. The rangers always looked after our kids, our six and their friends; there were so many kids, I don't know how they did it."

They walk back to the bath house where a picnic table is sheltered from the wind. Betty remembers more about the summers the family spent on the lake when Raymond was small.

"Jim could fish all he wanted and everyone else could hike, swim, play ball, row boats, fish, and do anything youngsters would love to spend long summer days doing. Some years, we camped on the site for an entire month, while Jim commuted back and forth to work each day, after his week off.

"The last time we came up to Deam's Lake with Raymond was in the summer after Carolyn left. He didn't want to come anymore. He said, 'Put a tent up in the yard,' and we'd spend nights out there but he wouldn't come to the lake anymore. Hindsight says the fun he had at Deam's Lake wasn't there any more with just Jim and Raymond and me. He had fun because of the kids. And they would take him around places. When we went that summer after Carolyn was gone to California, it was over. That was it for him."

The warmth and connectedness, the generous acceptance and hospitality and the humor and playfulness of Raymond's family made them the strong container for who Raymond was and what he needed in order to do well. Not every family has the confidence and depth of generosity to make life a positive process for a person with the needs that Raymond had. Gerald, Raymond's brother, put it this way:

"When we were young Mom and Dad told us, 'This is your brother for better or worse, and you've got to help take care of him.'

"They made us understand that he is a part of our family whether he is different or not. I don't know in other families if they key in on that child and say, 'He is a part of your family and you have to help him or her grow and be a better person,' or, I would say there are probably some families where parents shun their disabled child. That would be very tough on that child.

"Raymond was fortunate enough to be born into a family that accepted him. It changed our whole mind set. We never saw him as a burden. I never felt that from any of my siblings. As we grew up we were always told, 'You are not going to inherit anything; when we pass away the money will go to take care of Raymond.'

"We all accepted that with love, never a cross word or thought. We didn't feel cheated. We were fortunate enough to be 'complete.' We should go out and make it happen.

"Our whole family dynamics around Raymond made it work. I hope it's not rare. That would be sad. If only the parents would understand what type of life their child could have. It's not going to be an easy road; it wasn't for Mom and it wasn't for Dad, and for Mom it was real hard. But they stuck it through and Raymond had a good life."

Chapter 7

Family Supports

Some states have been moving through legislation and training toward a consumer-and-family directed approach to caring for people with disabilities. For a family like Raymond's this means a lot of hard work and diligent perseverance, but it is do-able for people with the energy and imagination and people-orientation that Betty and her family have. Many of us in Raymond's group feel that this is the ideal way to build a life for any family member, and certainly for one who needs the kinds of supports from the people around him that Raymond needed. But despite Gerald's hope, it is still quite rare.

We have many concerns about people without family supports who are living in institutions or in marginal situations in the community where there is minimal monitoring of a person's circumstances by impartial advocates or by a comprehensive care agency.

Some states are encouraging agencies working with people with disabilities to find individuals willing to volunteer to oversee and provide family-like supports to their clients. Like Carolyn with Clinton, a volunteer would step in to be "family" when the individual's family is unable to provide this care, or there is no family.

Julie recalls efforts in Kentucky that continue in support of community living for people with disabilities.

"In 2002 I worked with a grant program to recruit and encourage new volunteers to work as family supporters. Called Real Choices, this pilot state program would allow individuals to live safely in communities with a volunteer monitoring and supporting their living. I was exceedingly disappointed, in that year, at the few recruits we were able to find interested in becoming an advocate and monitor for the people who were in the pilot program. There will need to be an ongoing and powerful effort to interest people in offering such a service to others in their communities. Citizen Advocacy has been finding volunteers for many years who make this kind of commitment, but the numbers of volunteers have never met the numbers of individuals who need such support."

In Kentucky, in the summer of 2005, trainers went around the state to teach family

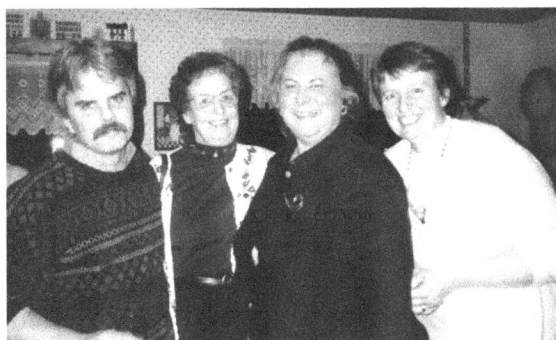

Milton Tyree, Betty Atherton, Nancy Bruccheri and Julie Cole at a meeting at Betty's house.

members about a similar pilot program, Consumer Directed Options*, for service program direction managed by the individual or by a family member or volunteer. This is an option under Supports for Community Living, part of the Medicaid Waiver in Kentucky allowing people to live outside of institutional settings. Ideally it would be the state's way of funding and overseeing similar self-chosen services like Raymond's family and team had set up for him. Like Raymond's team, people would work with an individual needing services to provide those services at the individual's choice. Raymond's team members believe that this is the ideal way that service provision be made, but it does require considerable commitment from "consumers" to direct their own lives. (For more information, see Chapter 14.)

You Make Me Nuts

Excerpt from poem –
December 29, 1997

Zibbet. Willie loved camping.
HE got a whiz bang out of it.
Too cold for me to go camping, Oh yeah.
Sleep in the bed tent, in it.
Sleep at night in the camper.
Deam lake. How is your swimming doing?
Daddy fishes.
Campfire. Smell it. Hot dogs. Roast the hot dogs.
Do you get one, Nancy?
Bout through.

Family supports beyond family

Even a family as warm and connected as Raymond's will have the usual developmental concerns as children grow and leave and make mistakes and make good decisions, and their parents age. For Raymond, things would be somewhat different than for his siblings who could go away to school, and then move to other places to work and start families. When it came time for Raymond to look at a life out on his own, it was a time for crisis. He wanted to leave, like any young man, but he did not want to leave since the anxiety he lived with would make such a drastic change unbearably frightening.

What could be done? Raymond's group was aware that this transition was going to take a lot of time and that there would have to be stages to go through to prepare Raymond for the difference that living more on his own would be. The first steps involved Raymond meeting new friends, like Milton and Chuck. Later Tony and Jim served to make Raymond's day a richer, more interesting experience.

When tension at home became difficult for everyone, and Raymond's day away became the best time for him and his family, the group looked into extending that supported day spent with Jim Schrecker and others into evening, with a view to using the time for training in more skills for independence. After some searching and recruitment efforts, Owen McWilliams was contacted through the Southern Baptist Seminary. Raymond spent evenings with the McWilliams family from 1995 to 1998, and the family lived briefly in Raymond's duplex when he first moved there, making that transition much smoother.

Owen shared these thoughts with the group:

"I cannot say that I brought any particular skill to working with Raymond. I really think that it was all just 'chemistry.' Raymond and I just hit it off from the 'git-go.' We both like to hang out; we both like to run around in the car; we both like witty banter. We were just a good match. It was one of those fortunate things that no one could have seen going in. Just luck.

From left, Betty Atherton, Tim Estes, Milton Tyree, Linda McAuliffe, Raymond, and Owen and Julie McWilliams at the Rudyard Kipling.

"Nevertheless, I am proud of the fact that in all my years of working with Raymond, there was never a single incident where Raymond felt the need to become upset. The closest we ever came was one incident fairly early on when Raymond was spending the week with Julie and me because home was too stressful for him. On this occasion Raymond was in the middle of watching 'Jeopardy' when the electricity went out. Anyone who knows him knows that this was a particularly difficult combination of stressors for Raymond. His reaction was to begin to yell out and pound on the wall. When he did this I simply said to him, 'Raymond, I know that you are upset, and I don't mind if you holler, but I don't want you to hit on my walls.' Raymond immediately stopped both yelling and hitting, and had no further problem, even though I had to go into the basement of the building to figure out the problem, leaving Raymond with Julie.

"Raymond always liked Julie even more than he did me. He loved to help her clean up the apartment for the brief time he came over to be with her during the day. He even enjoyed going on walks with her, which was one activity that I was told early on that he hated doing.

"That brings up a good point. I never tried to go for walks with Raymond because I was told that he hated walks. Come to find out, that wasn't true at all. I think that care should be taken in putting Raymond in a box, especially in telling people who work with him what to expect or not expect. I especially think that planting the idea in the minds of those who will spend time with Raymond that his 'explosions' are inevitable only creates 'self fulfilling prophecy.' I know for a fact that they do not have to be inevitable.

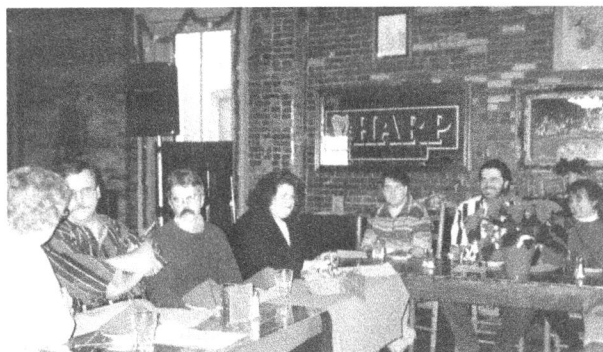

"It always struck me as funny that I could arrive at Raymond's to find him being restrained by someone, say to him 'Are you ready to go?' and see him hop up, come with me, and act no differently than on any other day."

I Love You

Excerpt from poem –
January 22, 1997

Me, I love you.
I love my mother.
And Dad.
I love my Dad.
I am sitting in the couch.
I am watching TV.
I am watching news.
It is on Channel 3
Scary movie.
Don't get me wrong, Nancy.
I be happy with it.
I broke the big screen TV.
It fell. It broke.
Knocked the end table over.
Knocked the phone over.
The TV where the couch is.
Snowman.
Making snow.
Rain.
Getting rain, too?
Go Away, the rain.
The sun came out.
Your's come out too?
Come back another day.
Wash the windows.
Watch the sunset. Moon.
In the sky.

Chapter 8

Key Chains

More invitations to outside support

In Raymond's new bedroom, as you look in the door, is a large board fastened to the right wall. On that board are hundreds of key chains of all kinds, shapes, colors, and sizes. There are cartoon animals and real animals, team insignia, slogan buttons, little flashlights, state-shaped cutouts and innumerable more types. They are Raymond's favorite collection, seconded only by his Pepsi paraphernalia collection and his budding assortment of M&M items. But the key chains are his pride and joy. He likes to invite people into his room to look at them.

Betty would take Raymond and go out to yard sales when he was little and look for lots of things, but Raymond chose key chains as his special interest.

"Raymond got a key chain that my mom gave to him. He thought that key chain was so important. We started to go to yard sales, really, before he stopped going to school. It went on a long time. We'd go to a sale and he would walk around every table and say, 'Any key chains?' And if there weren't any key chains, he was ready to go. People would want to give him key chains, and I said no, he has to pay for it. I wouldn't pay a dollar for one unless it was really special. I didn't usually see anything special. He bought a lot of them for a nickel. It was surprising how some of them he would just leave, and others he liked and would buy. He could tell you who gave him what key chain. His Daddy said, 'You want me to make you a board to hang them up?' Raymond really liked that. I know he got a few key chains from the members of the group. And that still meant something to him. Then Linda J. went overboard. She would bring bunches of them every time she came to visit. It got to be too much. Raymond would say, 'Linda, I don't want no more. Don't bring no more.' That's Linda, too. That took care of that.

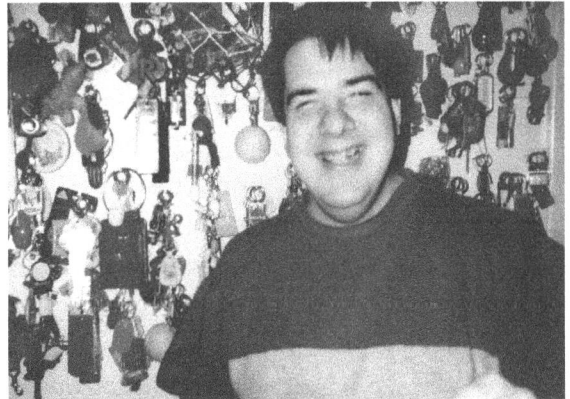

Raymond with his key chain collection.

"I have them all boxed up. I don't know what you would do with them, but I know I can't get rid of them."

Tim Estes mused, "We wished we could figure out some key to what was causing certain things with Raymond. It may have been Herb Lovett who said, 'You know there may not be this key.' The desire to have this key with everybody is kind of a mechanistic way of thinking. If you can find that one problem then you can medicate it or we can excise it or do whatever. It comes back to the desire to fix the person. After a lot of struggling with different things that happened with Raymond, I think it was a temptation for all of us to come back to that. We can talk about a lot of different things but we may not find that one thing that will fix this problem. That's what we have to live with."

There was a constant undercurrent of wanting to find the key. We humans are very susceptible to the urge to find gestalts, patterns. We want to solve the mystery, to hold the answer in a controllable package. Raymond couldn't help with his friends' need to know why, and they worked hard to just let Raymond be who he was. But now and again the group would succumb to the need to find out. And others would be brought in to consult, to observe, to help figure things out for Raymond's best outcome.

In 1993 Raymond's family and friends were particularly concerned about the health of his grandmother. His reaction to his beloved grandfather's death left Betty nearly trapped in the home. For about three weeks he kept asking for him to come back. After that he acted out about anything and everything. It went on for more than two years. After about two years, Betty asked Dr. Roth how long one grieves. He said, "I don't know. Some do for a lifetime."

Raymond became terrified that if Betty or Jim went out, they wouldn't come back. And he let them know how he felt. The group talked about this and what might be done. Someone suggested that Raymond talk with Renelle Grubbs, a Seven Counties Services counselor who specialized in grief and domestic disturbance. Carol Stuecker from Project Neighbor suggested a movie about grief, like *All Dogs Go to Heaven*. Maybe an art therapist* that she knew of in the neighborhood could help Raymond express his concerns. Some of the group members reviewed the movie and didn't feel it was the best choice for Raymond. Carol contacted Julie Cole, who agreed to meet with Raymond to do art and perhaps deal with grief issues over time. Betty hoped that art therapy would give Raymond another way to express his feelings.

Art therapy

"On a pleasant sunny November day I waited by the door of our little office building, formerly the manse for the Lutheran church on the corner of my street. I looked out as a little bright red sports car drove up. Two large men climbed out of the tiny car, and headed up the front walk. One was a little shorter with lighter thinning hair and a ready smile. The other man was taller with dark short hair and a soft, rounded face. He looked down and walked with some hesitation. They came in and Jim Schrecker introduced me to his friend Raymond Atherton. I invited them up the stairs to my office. As he carefully climbed the stairs, Raymond looked down and did not make any kind of eye contact. He rarely spoke during our first meeting.

"I had decided to use this time to see what Raymond's attention span could be, and to feel out how he'd react to drawing and making things. I often do this on a first visit, to get an idea of what the person will enjoy, and how he might best benefit from art therapy. When I offered Raymond a small selection of colorful markers, I could tell that introducing any new materials would be a serious source of anxiety. Although I had been called before what Raymond occasionally yelled out, I realized that his ninety-decibel 'Bitch' was not directed at me, but at the difficult experience of doing something or touching something new and unfamiliar. I set up all our meetings after the first one so that Raymond would meet just one new experience in the visit. I worked toward making the newness be a part of a previously safe material or activity. Over time, Raymond became relatively comfortable with art materials and less afraid of glues or paints, which seemed uncontrollable to him. Raymond counted on routine, as we all do, to help him get past the scariest parts of his day.

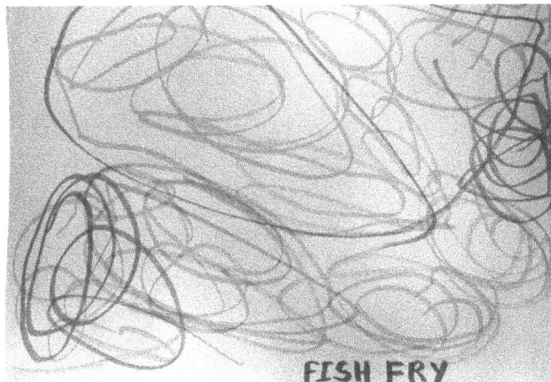

Raymond's painting "Fish Fry."

"Presented with large paper and the nice bright markers, Raymond began to make his pictures. While his drawings may have been graphically similar in development to a pre-schooler's, they had a lot of zest and personality and charm. He would tend to draw one shape over and over, but was quite happy to move on when given an appropriate prompt. He drew trees, long green and brown figures, but without branches or roots. When I asked Raymond to draw his home, he drew what appeared at first to be three figures, but a second look and a prompt from Jim made me realize he had signed his name, RAY. What an interesting response.

"When I asked if he would like to draw a person, he made a loopy set of circles.

"'Who is that?'

"'Jim.'

"'Does Jim have eyes?'

"Raymond looks at Jim, who smiles. Raymond smiles and laughs, 'Yeah.' In go two circles. He then adds another circle for a mouth.

"Next he did some free drawings making large loopy circles. 'This is money,' he suggested. Jim said that Raymond liked to write notes to send to his Group friends when he announced meetings. So Raymond drew a note and signed his name. He finished up by drawing cookies to serve at the meeting. Raymond is ever the generous host.

"I asked Raymond if he wanted to come back and meet with me again. He shouted,

'Bitch!' Then he said he would like to come back and do more art work. So we set a time for a few weeks away.

"At first the longer time between visits helped Raymond to get used to the idea of coming. After the first year, Raymond visited about every other week for around five years. His visits became fun times for Raymond, his variable companion for the day, and for me. And he dictated a lot of poems during his later visits. These served as keys to many of his inner thoughts, making them more available to his family and friends. This brought his conversation out of the safety of often-repeated questions into useful and humorous repartee.

"Raymond enjoyed doing all sorts of art work, and doing reading readiness exercises, but his two favorite things at 'art class' were painting and conversation. He painted with great abandon and delight, and often would say, 'This is relaxing.' Our conversations and jokes eventually broadened into the dictated poems, which were really his side of vigorous exchanges of questions and answers and a lot of laughter. One day after some side-splitting laughs between Raymond, Nancy, and me, Raymond leaned over and touched my hand and said, 'I love you, Julie.' Then he turned to Nancy and said he loved her, too. And we knew he meant it."

After Raymond had been doing art therapy sessions, the group began to wonder if it might be possible for him to learn to read. Being able to read would give him a new set of job skills that might open doors for him. Betty mentioned that he had some success with his letters at Tulley. One teacher there, Ms. Accordino, recognized Raymond's innate intelligence and worked hard with him to recognize letters and understand words.

The group discussed this at several meetings, and decided to bring in Jayne Miller who was an expert at reading instruction for people with learning disabilities, and who was familiar with facilitated communication.* Jayne spent several meetings with Raymond. While working with him she decided that he probably would have difficulty tracking letters enough to make words into sentences. Julie had worked a lot with Raymond on word recognition and realized that he relied as much on images as on letter/sound construction of words. He loved brand names and could tell many brands simply by recognizing the logo, or the colors of the wrapper.

Jayne Miller developed a scrapbook that Raymond could use to help him when he met new people. Together they developed pages that described the people that were important to him; the places that he frequented, or wanted to; the activities that he enjoyed. Julie and Raymond added a lot of word recognition pages to the scrapbook which he could use to tell people more about what he was thinking. Raymond's poems that he dictated also went into his scrapbook.

A Visit from Herb Lovett

There were times when things would seem to feel so static for Raymond. Nothing seemed to be changing and his anxieties would escalate. His behavior became more disruptive and uncomfortable and the group would have to find new supports for him.

At one point they decided to ask Herb Lovett, the psychologist from Boston, to visit Raymond and give him and his support group suggestions for more effective communication, or again, keys to what was going on with Raymond.

Milton and Hope contacted Dr. Lovett. Hope had known him before through his work with other individuals. Julie had met Dr. Lovett at a Seven Counties Conference that Jeff Strully had coordinated some years before. She also felt that if anyone could really listen to Raymond, Herb could.

Dr. Lovett's books, the obviously academic *Cognitive Counseling For Persons With Special Needs: Adapting Behavioral Approaches to the Social Context* (New York: Praeger, 1985), and his more accessible *Learning to Listen* (Baltimore: Paul H. Brookes, 1998), opened many people's eyes and ears to the simple real awareness needed to comprehend the needs and subtle communication of people with communication and cognitive disabilities.

Dr. Lovett's visit was scheduled for March 17, 1996. The day was planned like a bank heist, with everyone's location known at every moment throughout the day, for ease of transportation and to cause Raymond the least possible stress. The whole group was determined to make the most of Dr. Lovett's time and expertise.

Nancy sent out a schedule so everyone would be aware of times and synchronize their watches.

9:00-9:45 – Group members will meet at Raymond's to prepare for day. Betty, Nancy, Milton, and Hope signed up. Hope will bring Herb. Tim and Raymond will go to breakfast.

9:45 -10:45 – Herb, Raymond, and Jim will spend community time.

11:00 12:00   Raymond, Nancy, and Herb will meet with Julie for observation of Ray's art work.

12:00 – Hope, Linda, and Raymond meet at Julie's and go to lunch. Nancy takes Herb to the Athertons' for lunch with family.

1:30 to 4:00 – Group meets at Atherton house. Ray will be there or not as seems appropriate.

Raymond was nervous, having a new person in his orbit. He handled things pretty well through the long day. It all started with breakfast at Betty's. Over his toast and juice Herb met Raymond and got to know him in a neutral and non-threatening environment. Then part of the team met with Herb to give him the day plan, and

Raymond went out for the first part of his usual day with Tim, to ease the tension a bit with some comfortable routine.

At eleven Raymond had his art session. Herb again met Raymond at Julie's studio/office. She worked for and shared office space with The Advocado Press, a publisher of books and a magazine on civil rights for people with disabilities. Julie was upstairs and looked out as Dr. Lovett and Nancy and Raymond arrived. Herb pointed at the sign in front of the building. From the window Julie laughed as she saw Herb say, 'Wow, this is the Advocado Press.' Dr. Lovett was familiar with and enjoyed the Press' signature magazine, then called *The Disability Rag* (archived online as *Ragged Edge* at www.advocadopress.org). So that made Herb feel more at home.

Julie tells about the session:

"I ran downstairs and Nancy reintroduced me to Dr. Lovett. At the conference where I first met him I was enormously impressed by Herb's fresh way of approaching relationships with people with disabilities. His way consisted of being with people with disabilities exactly the same way you would be with anyone else. This might sound easy, but try it with all your cultural prejudices and personal discomforts blocking the way and see how tricky it can be. Dr. Lovett's latest book at the time he met Raymond was *Learning to Listen.* It was a subtly brilliant book about ways that we miss the obvious in people we regard as different.

"Herb asked Raymond if it would be all right if he sat in while Raymond had his art lesson. Raymond was tense, but not disturbed enough to change his behavior in Herb's presence. But there was a subtle difference in his demeanor: more guarded and less ebullient. We started with collage-illustrated sentences. At each visit at this time, Raymond was building word recognition by reading simple words illustrated with photo images, usually cut from magazines and arranged in a collage/rebus format. In a slightly more hesitant manner than usual Raymond read the illustrated phrases, 'The Men Ride Horses; The Man Hugs the Boy; The Man Winds the Watch; and What Time Is It?' Raymond recognized Boy, Watch, Horses, and Time. Dr. Lovett watched quietly from a chair across the room.

"We began to glue more collages to identify new words and pictures. Gluing had taken time for Raymond to get used to. But by this session he was relatively comfortable and quick about doing the gluing, especially as long as his trusty red towel was right at his hand for a quick wipe.

"After the word portion of the work, Raymond was excited to get into finger painting. This formerly deeply threatening activity was now a relaxing and pleasurable process. Raymond didn't use his fingers; that would have been more than one could ask. He instead used a small damp sponge to move paint. This day he moved the paint on the heavy bristol board so briskly that very little paint was being left on the paper. There was not enough paint to press effective prints from the bristol board onto newsprint sheets. So attention was focused on the board itself. Raymond was using acrylic reds in different hues. He used the sponge to layer different reds over each other all over the paper. He completed it to his satisfaction and called the painting, 'Fine.' He offered it to Herb as a gift. Herb accepted it graciously and told Raymond the painting reminded him of the work of a Boston artist named Philip Guston. He also has layered colors in paintings.

"After Raymond completed his art work, Herb said that he felt what Raymond was doing could be called 'facilitated art,' and Raymond seemed pleased about this."

After art, Raymond went out to have a late lunch with Jim while the group met with Dr. Lovett to listen to what he was learning about Raymond's situation.

Herb said that he wouldn't differ from a "diagnosis" of pervasive developmental disorder.* When group members pressed him, he said it was a blanket label that described only that Raymond had always had the perceptual and communication problems that made things different for him. He encouraged the group to have some tests done by a neuropsychologist to see what kinds of input-output differences Raymond had so we could make our communication with him the best it could be. Herb didn't have a magic solution for what made Raymond so anxious and prone to very loud comments and "moving furniture."

He further encouraged us to look into facilitated communication, since the facilitated art seemed to work so well for Raymond. He said that structured movement would be a good thing to add to Raymond's art therapy.

He said that what the group is doing, really trying to listen to and work with Raymond's desires in his life, is the best for the long term outcome for Raymond and his plans.

Best for the group was Herb's promise that we could bug him anytime with questions and feedback, and he would continue to share with us.

During the same month that Dr. Lovett visited Raymond, Jo Ann Boyle, who had organized the first meetings for Raymond's group, was invited to revisit for an "update" planning session with the whole group. She picked up the markers and went to work. After the meeting she returned to St. Louis and sent Raymond this letter about her view from close up and a distance:

Mar. 15, 1996
Dear Raymond,

Thank you for the wonderful fellowship together last week. I was excited to be invited back to be a part of your group. Friends like you are not to be taken for granted in this world today. I received such warm love from you, after hiding in St. Louis for three years, that I was reminded of what realness is all about. It was refreshing.

Raymond, you look great. I sensed a joy with you, that reminds me of those brief moments on Christmas morning when you see someone you love open the gift you gave them with pure excitement and anticipation, and then realizing that their greatest dream was fulfilled. The only difference in you is that your joy seems to be bigger than any joy connected with a gift that you receive at Christmas. Your joy is connected to something that can't fit into a box . . . and something that doesn't wear out or get lost, or get used up. It was revealing to me to see that, and I just need to thank you for giving me a glimpse into your life again, so I could take a fresh glimpse into mine.

Well, share with everyone in the group that I finally got my paperwork done. They know me too well, and know that I don't like paperwork and stuff. I think they were afraid that I wasn't ever going to do it. You don't need to tell them that if it was anyone else but you, I probably would not have done it. I would like the group to still think that I am reputable.

You have a great set of people around you. I thank God for that. As you know, everyone put their heads together, with your input, to see what life for you might look like in the future. I hope this letter explains some of the key points that were birthed from that time together. Some of this is just my "peanut butter" input keeping the peas on the knife, if you know what I mean. I filled in some blanks with my opinion and thoughts, so please forgive me, Raymond, if you don't approve. Just tell the group you think I'm off my rocker, and they'll listen to you.

Everything good that's going to happen will require divine patience and careful building. Step by step. We know that there is a great foundation in your life, not only in the people you know but in the changes that you have made for yourself. Together with you and your friends and family, things can happen. Everyone just needs to do their part. Sometimes it seems like you work really hard and nothing happens. Things may even seem worse. Most people would give up, quitting altogether, or changing their plan to an easier one to complete. I'm glad that you are surrounded by a lot of people who know how to walk in the dark without giving up. I'm glad that your friends and family know how to press forward, never being content, so that greater things can be revealed for you. With all of that said, let me review "THE PLAN."

"The Plan" seems pretty simple and obvious really. It's making it happen where the intricacy of our plan is revealed. Because of that, I've drawn out a chart to help Nancy and other folks who help steer the ship have a reference. This is what sounded good to you, Raymond:

1. Your own place.

2. Your own stuff.

3. More friends and people to meet.

4. More interesting things to do.

Here are a few things that everyone else threw in, because it made sense to them:

1. Nurture responsibility.

2. A full routine . . . maybe a job.

3. More ways to say what's on your mind, to open more doors for things to happen.

It made sense to me too, that's why I put it in. Just remember though: you're the boss, so keep us honest.

I suppose that I sensed that the real theme is "What's in store?" What will the next level of dreaming bring? What about Raymond beyond Betty, or otherwise referred to as Raymond B.B. Well, Raymond, there will be lots more meetings for you. People will want to talk to you about what you think about things. Just be patient and have fun with them. Everyone loves you a lot.

Jo Ann looked at what the group had done so far, and made some solid recommendations for movement in the future. She put these in a letter to the group that Raymond shared with everyone. She thanked everyone for their patience and complimented the group on their ongoing support of Raymond and his family.

"I'm seeing Raymond's planning meeting come to a new level," Jo Ann shared.

"In four years (or was it five), some great things have happened for Raymond. When we had our first meeting, Raymond wasn't keen on leaving home; didn't encourage people visiting; rarely moved from his couch, and continually watched TV. He would impulsively scream out when agitated, and tolerated people and activities with little patience on his part.

"Looking at Ray now, he appears to be a different person than before. He's been given an opportunity to develop trust and love for people other than his family. He's been given a forum to explore and become outwardly the person he has always been inwardly."

Jo Ann outlined what she felt the group had learned from Raymond since they started meeting:

"Raymond is a delightful, warm person. His world CAN be expanded.

"He can gain some control of his outbreaks. He cares and wants to please people.

"People care and make commitments to Raymond and his family that are accountable."

Jo Ann goes on to note the following things that had happened for Raymond since he had been supported by the circle in new ways.

"His circle of friends has expanded from Jennie to the many who attend his fish fry. His scope has expanded from his couch to the outside world; his outside world has expanded from the Highlands and St. Matthews to wherever he and Jim cruise in Jim's convertible. We know Raymond has feelings. We are glad he is beginning to express his inward self through his time in art therapy. There is so much to learn.

"In summary our expectations for Raymond were exceeded beyond our WILD-EST imagination. This outcome represents reaching level one in Raymond's life."

Never one to stop at success, Jo Ann urged the group to press on with continued realization of Raymond's goals. She pushed the ideas on to a second level

"Level Two introduces new challenges, bigger dreams, and tougher questions to solve. I encourage you as Raymond's friends to approach this time in his life with a bigger view of potential resources for Raymond. Really stretch your comfort zone with new ideas about what will work for Raymond. Try new things. Always encourage his growth beyond the boundaries he sets for himself. Encourage more risk taking."

But she curbed the eagerness a bit by reminding the group, "It may mean moving slower toward the goals in mind. It may mean a lot of small setbacks.

"The ultimate goal is the important one: Raymond's independence so that Betty won't have to provide the extensive primary care that she is currently managing. It's OK to time Raymond's success so that Betty may enjoy his new life and independence."

So. Jo Ann reassured the group, "The original goals have been met."

But she challenged the group to push on, "Remembering that our new destination is for Raymond to be established.

"This will require new roles.

"It will require planning for long term stability.

"It will require an immense amount of support for and by everyone involved.

"People will get discouraged; but keep looking to the result intended.

"Attempt smaller goals, and involve more people in that goal for the energy, the creativity, and the support.

"There is no reason to keep Raymond from having the life typical to others his age."

Jo Ann encouraged the group to keep meetings to brief, task-oriented gatherings. She felt that a short agenda would support more accomplishment. Cover specifics. Break into subgroups to deal with specific issues and have those smaller groups report back to the large meeting.

"For example, a subgroup of Betty, Jim, Owen, and Nancy may meet to develop strategies for introducing Raymond to new people.

"Regardless of how the meetings are orchestrated, the important thing is to stay focused and on task, and always consult and get input and feedback from Raymond. But everyone knows that better than me."

Jo Ann's encouragement and her objective overview of the initial years of work by the group on Raymond's behalf made it easier for the group to see accomplishments.

With that clearer picture the movement forward also seemed easier to envision.

Input from Jo Ann, John O'Brien, Wade Hitzig, Herb Lovett, and others broadened the group's perspective, and provided energy for the journey ahead. These visits with experts in developmental disability couldn't provide the magic key that the group had only half hoped for. But asking and receiving feedback added batteries to the tiny flashlight as the group continued moving through the cave of unknown solutions. And the confidence and creativity stimulated by Jo Ann's feedback gave the group impetus to keep on pushing and moving ahead. As Jo Ann pointed out, it was getting to know Raymond as he is and working with him where he was that made the group's efforts most worthwhile.

Chapter 9

Antennae –
Raymond Being Himself

I Love You

December 5, 1996

I'M good.
I am good for a prize.
Be happy
The answering machine is loud.
Answer the phone call.
Jim's phone call.
To Hope.
To Terry.
I live here.
In the bathroom.
I am in a good mood today.
I be happy.
I am not grumpy anymore.
Did you take the car to the VET?
You love me.
Don't cancel me Nancy.
The garbage.
The garbage collection.
Don't miss the meeting, Nancy.
You want to go, Julie?
Wednesday.
To the Mexican Restaurant.
El Napolito. You Going?
I am happy in my room.

My TV.

It's on the table.

I want an antenna.

Don't miss the meeting, Nancy.

You going to try to be there?

Mom and I are going shopping on Friday.

We are looking at TVs.

A 42-inch TV.

You want to see it, Nancy?

You want to go, Julie?

Fine.

What am I going to do over at Denise's?

Baking cookies.

I love you, Nancy. You're sweet.

The Radio Shack is a little busier than usual. The tall sturdy sales clerk is watching the curious man who comes in with a tape recorder and records audio from the radios and TVs in the back display area. The salesman is wondering if this taping is illegal or if it is just for personal use and not an issue. But he just doesn't know. He has sometimes fantasized that the small dark-haired man might be a very inept spy from some distant land who is either trying to learn the language or is mistakenly sending these odd taped missives back home. He's just another one of the characters that come in to the Shack.

The door opens again and a lady with dark and silver curly hair comes in hurriedly. She runs back and is looking through TV antennas, "rabbit ears," and adaptors. The quiet young salesman approaches her. In his soft, almost swallowed voice he says, "Ma'm, is there anything I could help you with?"

"Oh, yes. I need a few antenna connector things real quick. You know those things that go between the TV and the rabbit ears." She answers in a deep smoky voice with a gentle drawl behind it.

It wasn't quite what he expected, but kind of went along with the rest of the day. So he helped her find the RF adaptors that she felt would be compatible with the TVs she needed them for. She said she'd like a dozen.

"A dozen?! Watch a lot of TV?" He couldn't help himself from asking facetiously.

"Well, no. But my son does. He has a few TVs in his room. And the antennas tend to get broken a lot, unh huh."

She paid the young man, and he watched her as she ran back out to her car and sped off. As he turned and saw the man who'd been taping rush out the door with his little recorder, he wondered what a person does to break a lot of antennas.

"My son was working at Radio Shack at this time," Julie remarked "and he came home and told us about this lady who came in to buy TV antennas in multiples. It didn't take long for me to figure out that this was my friend Betty."

Betty laughed at the coincidence and shared more about Raymond and his televisions.

"When Raymond would 'move furniture' during his tense and dark times, he occasionally threw his televisions. These TVs were Raymond's great occupation and consolation. For a number of years we would replace these, but only one at Christmas time. So Raymond knew that if he threw and broke a TV that he would not get a replacement until Christmas."

Often in between getting new TVs, Raymond ripped off antennas and threw them. Betty needed to have a supply on hand in order to fix the TVs for Raymond. Raymond would talk about his anticipated Christmas television for weeks before the holiday.

"Santa's going to bring a TV. Going to H.H. Gregg to look at them. I'm going to be waiting, waiting at the door. I'm going to be excited. I am going to be a happy man."

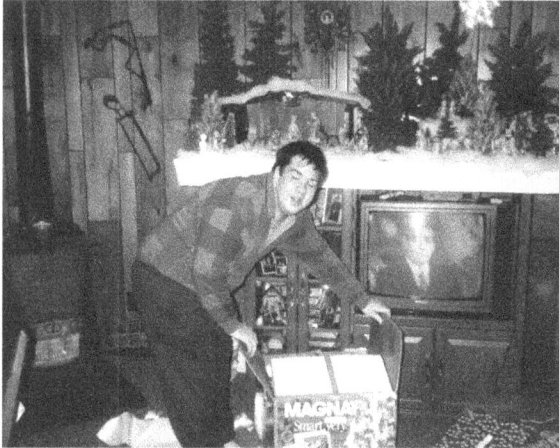

Raymond with a
Christmas TV.

Rain

It is raining today.
I watched it bloom in the sky.
It runs down my window.
I like to watch it run down my window.
It goes down the sidewalk, and into the ground.
It makes mushrooms grow.
It pours down.
It washes the windows.
It doesn't say, "I don't do windows."
I bet you'll get a kick out of this one.
I'm not banging on the door.
I'm laughing.
I've got a smile on my face.
I am happy. Happy.
I threw a fit last night.

It made me sad.
I know I'll get well.
I shut the door to my bedroom easy.
It made me happy.
I cried about a chair.
I did not break the door.
I was sad, and I was happy.
There was nothing on the TV.
That made me happy, yeah.
I like to watch "Another World."
It is a soap opera.
Husband watch it? No?
I got a haircut.
I liked it.
The barber shop cut it. It was fun.
The rain has quit.
The lights go off.
It makes me happy when the lights go back on.
The lights go out. It makes me sad.
I light a candle . . .

Besides having a very whimsical sense of humor, and a poignant sense of his own anxiety, Raymond endeared himself to us by showing many signs of clairvoyance of sorts, or a kind of E.S.P. that was Raymond's own. No one really wanted to hear him say, "How's your car?" Experience told us this could mean that your brakes or transmission were about to go, or as in one person's case, the door would fall off. This ability to "see" also included appliances and office equipment.

Alex, who spent days with Raymond, told Betty that Raymond would tell him things. "Alex, you didn't take the garbage out," Raymond would admonish Alex, although no discussion about garbage or what Alex had done before coming to visit Raymond had occurred.

"You left your keys in the car again," Raymond would tell the unaware Alex perhaps emphasizing the "again" just to get Alex's goat a little bit.

When Julie moved into a new art therapy studio, Raymond seemed right at home the first day. He was sitting with Nancy and talking with Julie in the studio area. He asked how the new computer was doing. The computer was in a separate office, and he had never seen it or been told about it.

 Another time he came in for an art class wearing a shirt with a picture on it nearly identical to the seascape that was waiting for him to work on. He liked the juxtaposition of the similar pictures.

Several times in the context of his art session, or at meetings, Raymond would announce what would happen. "Nancy is going to the bathroom now." Nancy would look at Julie with a very wide-eyed grin, shake her head and get up to leave the room. At other times he would say, "Nancy has something important to say to you." Then he would get up and go take a restroom break, leaving Nancy to tell Julie what Nancy didn't know he was aware of.

Here is a section of art therapy notes for April 8, 1997:

> Raymond is bringing a lot of interest to our sessions. From our first visits together to now, the difference in the amount of talking he does is remarkable. We began with leisurely and extensive conversation about things that interest him. He is very careful to engage by asking everything that might be of interest to you. He asks about your nourishment, your special friends and relatives and their situations, your daily schedule, family's schedules, and then those eerie clairvoyant questions about things that are malfunctioning in your life. 'How's your freezer?'
>
> He asked that today, and my freezer is really "on the fritz," one of Raymond's favorite expressions.

Julie found these moments fascinating and felt they were an important part of Raymond's communication with others. She writes, "On one of these occasions I asked Raymond about how he knew these things. He acknowledged that he did know, but didn't know how it happens."

Raymond knew many things but wasn't always capable of accessing them and getting others to understand.

After Raymond moved into the duplex, and his brother Gerald moved in downstairs, they spent a lot of time together in the new house.

"Raymond surprised me a lot," Gerald remembers.

"When a person is like Raymond, you don't really know what he knows. To give you an example of what he taught me, I never really thought much on how people learned. We were watching 'Jeopardy' together and he popped the answer out of the blue before the guy on the show did, and I said, 'Raymond?! How did you know that?' And he says, 'I'm smart.' and I said, 'No way you could know that!' And I was like tripping out and I got to thinking, 'How did he know that answer?' Maybe it was a rerun."

Gerald speculated about what makes people learn. He felt that repetition of actions and information was one way that we learn.

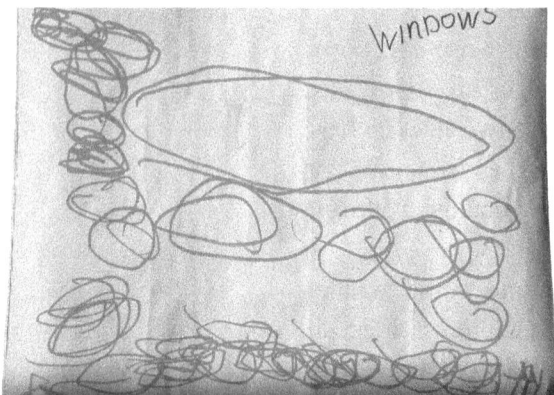

Raymond's painting "Windows."

"Raymond probably saw that 'Jeopardy' before once, maybe three times, I don't know. But it enlightened me. It was things like that that people who may never spend time with a person like him would never grasp. It was just that little block of some-thing he taught me. They would look at him and say he's handicapped or he's dumb. We can learn from people, maybe minute things. But the enlightenment I got from that, I was just blown away."

Gerald delighted in the surprises that his brother offered him, and the changes that he saw in him as he became more independent in his own apartment, upstairs from Gerald.

"I always took it for granted that Raymond never really read, but he showed me how much he understood the world around him. One evening we were driving around in my G-wagon and we pulled up behind a Toyota, he goes, 'Toyota.' And I thought, 'There is no way he could know that was a Toyota unless he could read that word.' And he told me, 'Yeah I can read, I just can't read like you do.'

"I didn't realize how much my brother grasped. I learned to read body language in how he would carry himself. He couldn't always say what he liked or disliked; it was more action and body language. He could say things, like 'I am so happy' and all that. But if he was angry or uncomfortable it was more act out, pick up things and throw them.

"You know I think Raymond, and people like Raymond, have so many turn-offs for so long that I could see how it would take time for them to trust anyone," Betty ob-served as we sat around her big table.

Tim supported her observation and added, "Thank God that Raymond was the assertive person that he was. When he said "no," it was partly because so many people had told him, 'You have to do this and you have to do it this way.'

"That's the way people get treated, especially people who are vulnerable in our society. They get told 'this is the way you have to do it.' His assertiveness got him re-jected by a lot of the system that was there supposedly for his support. When people gathered around him who said, 'We're going to accept Raymond and believe in what Raymond wants,' it gave them the opportunity to learn what Raymond really did want to do. Like, 'I don't want to be on this flight. I don't want to be on this elevator.' And he taught the lesson well. As offensive as that might have been to some people looking on, it was Raymond's way of saying, 'You're not going to make me be what you want me to be. You need to understand who I am.'"

There seem to be tacit cultural assumptions about people with disabilities, generaliza-tions that try to collect many diverse people into one group. The assumption is that these are people with disabilities who are intrinsically unhappy with who and how they are. But many people who live with all sorts of disabilities are simply who they are, and it is the perceptions and projections of others that make being that difficult.

In an article in the December 20, 2004 *New York Times*, reporter Amy Harmon shows how a group of young people describe this difficulty they experience from others, a difficulty they don't experience within themselves:

BOICEVILLE, N.Y. – Jack Thomas, a 10th grader at a school for autistic teenagers and an expert on the nation's roadways, tore himself away from his satellite map one recent recess period to critique a television program about the search for a cure for autism. "We don't have a disease," said Jack, echoing the opinion of the other 15 boys at the experimental Aspie School here in the Catskills. "So we can't be 'cured.' This is just the way we are. . . ."

The autistic activists say they want help, too, but would be far better off learning to use their autistic strengths to cope with their autistic impairments rather than pretending that either can be removed. Some autistic tics, like repetitive rocking and violent outbursts, they say, could be modulated more easily if an effort were made to understand their underlying message, rather than trying to train them away.

Other traits, like difficulty with eye contact, with grasping humor or with breaking from routines, might not require such huge corrective efforts on their part if people were simply more tolerant. . . . "We need acceptance about who we are and the way we are."

A neurological condition that can render standard forms of communication like tone of voice, facial expression and even spoken language unnatural and difficult to master, autism has traditionally been seen as a shell from which a normal child might one day emerge. But some advocates contend that autism is an integral part of their identities, much more like a skin than a shell, and not one they care to shed. . . .

The effort to cure autism, they say, is not like curing cancer, but like the efforts of a previous age to cure left-handedness. Some worry that in addition to troublesome interventions, the ultimate cure will be a genetic test to prevent autistic children from being born. That would be a loss, they say, not just for social tolerance but because autistics, with their obsessive attention to detail and eccentric perspective, can provide valuable insight and innovation. The neurologist Oliver Sacks, for instance, contends that Henry Cavendish, the 18th-century chemist who discovered hydrogen, was most likely autistic. . . . "Behaviors are so often attempts to communicate," said Jane Meyerding, an autistic woman who has a clerical job at the University of Washington and is a frequent contributor to the Autistic Advocacy e-mail discussion list. "When you snuff out the behaviors you snuff out the attempts to communicate." . . .

Terry Walker, 37, who has Asperger's syndrome, said he was not opposed to the concept of a cure for autism but he suggested that there was a pragmatic reason to look for other options.

"I don't think it's going to be easy to find," Mr. Walker said. "That's why I opt for changing the world around me; I think that does more long-term good."

Chapter 10

ReModeling –
Finding a Place

In 1998 Hope was serving the as family broker* and facilitator. Raymond was spending a lot of his afternoons and evenings with the McWilliams family. Things were uncomfortable at home, because Jim Atherton was very ill and Betty was taking care of him. This took her time away from Raymond and that made things difficult for him. He was anxious about being away. He was anxious about his Dad being sick.

The group meetings were taking on a feeling of urgency. Owen McWilliams frequently complained that everyone seemed to be just sitting still and things needed to be happening. Everybody was concerned about what sort of housing Raymond would find to best suit his needs. Everybody was also concerned about more subtle things. How will Raymond react to moving? How gradual should the moving process be? Raymond had expressed a few times that "I don't want my stuff moved." The group also worried about how much anxiety he would have to tolerate to make the transition. How much change could he cope with? How could the group help Raymond make this change more manageable?

Another worry was what kind of home Raymond could live in. Could other building occupants deal with his occasional noise and verbal outbursts? Would a landlord tolerate his "furniture moving" which occasionally led to wall or door damage?

At one of Raymond's meetings the pressure of Raymond's home situation and his interest in being outside the home prompted the group to get active about housing.

"We have this house up here on the paper, and we need to surround it with possibilities. Everyone make a suggestion for a way that we can look at and act on finding an alternative living situation for Raymond." Hope nudged the group for ideas.

"Betty and I have been looking at apartments in this area," Nancy offered. "There

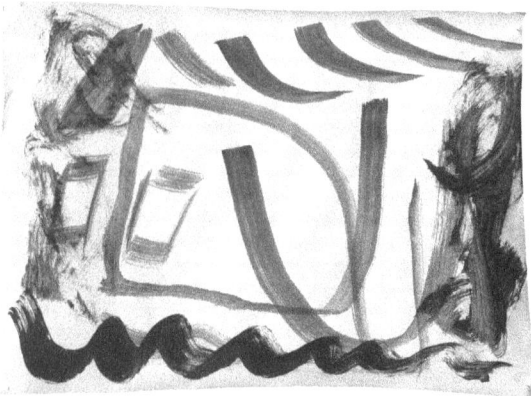

Raymond's painting "House."

was a four-plex, but we thought, what would people in the other apartments do when there might be noise from one apartment?"

"Well that is possible, but it can't be a total end to the idea of getting that sort of apartment," Hope says as she draws a little four-plex house off of a line from the big house on the sheet. "It would be important for Raymond to get to know his neighbors; to be a good neighbor, to visit around and share cookies, that kind of thing."

She draws in neighbors and people meeting people.

"Then if there are occasional noise issues, they might just shrug and say, 'There's Raymond.'"

"We talked to several Realtors about possibilities, but nothing has really presented itself that felt right." Betty says.

"At this time I really couldn't consider doing housekeeping at two different locations. Something else would have to happen so that wouldn't be the outcome."

Betty looked worn with all the caring she was doing for her ill husband and her mother, who regularly called on her for help. And of course even though Raymond at that time was spending nearly twelve hours a day out with Jim Schrecker, and Owen and Julie McWilliams, and doing some other activities, too, still Betty was with him through the night and got him up and going, and down and settled, morning and nights. She wondered if she could actually do all that would be necessary for her to get Raymond transitioned into another home.

Application to HUD*

Soon Hope found out that in three months she and her family would be moving to Wisconsin to Paul's new job. Hope felt a real sense of urgency and push, like time to make this "baby" come. She began to talk more to Realtors and apartment owners. Hope and Betty went to the Housing Authority* and applied for a Section 8* housing voucher. They found the office in the old nursing school building of the former Baptist Hospital.

Betty said, "When we went there, we found out that to get the voucher Raymond's home couldn't be a family-owned place. Of course we were thinking about the possibility of family purchasing a place for Raymond to rent. Hope really thinks on her feet. She said, 'Can we look at it this way?' We had to go to the higher ups to make it work."

Art Wasson of the Housing Authority agreed and said that Section 8 cannot apply to property owned by a family member except in some cases where disability is the issue. Since Raymond's disability made getting housing much more challenging, he qualified under this arrangement.

"Sometimes I think," mused Betty, "when you are in things like that, like I was, you don't see the forest for the trees. But from the outside you can see it better. Hope, as advocate, was more on the outside. She had more room to dicker, to explore all possibilities. I might have been more likely to hear one answer and not push for more.

"Those people in the HUD office sure could make you miserable. You had to go down an average of two or three times a year to apply and reapply. And if it wasn't right you had to re-do it."

Betty and Hope had to go to HUD several times. Betty was losing heart and getting discouraged. It seemed like so much work for so little return. It felt like just a lot of rejection, and there was no guarantee that Raymond would be able to get the voucher.

The estimated wait for Section 8 housing was three to four years in 2005. Betty and Hope were actually lucky to have applied when they did, in 1998. And if there was a property already available for Raymond to live in, the process would be that much easier.

Family involvement

Meanwhile, Raymond's sister Carolyn and her husband, Syd, had been talking about what could be done to provide a nice home for Raymond. When Raymond's father died at the end of May 1998 that shifted everyone's sense of urgency.

One day that summer Syd called Carolyn and asked her to come to look at a place. It was a charming duplex with potential for two-bedroom apartments down and up. The apartments had a connecting stairway that opened into the side yard. The stairway made for easy access to both apartments from inside, but afforded privacy for each space with separate interior doors. The house was only a few blocks from Carolyn and Syd's home. It was on a well-traveled suburban street with two churches across the street and a nice-sized yard in front and back.

Carolyn recalled it this way. "There was a duplex for sale. It wasn't like we were going out and looking for anything. Syd just drove by and looked at it. It could have been that he was looking at it for rental property in general and not so much for Raymond.

"We bought it and Mom offered to help work on it and it just became The Project. With Raymond coming over we had to have a place for him to sit and a TV and some Pepsis on hand. So Raymond got involved and excited with the progress. We kept saying what a cute little house it is, and Raymond came to love it just as much as we did. It just evolved and happened. That was real exciting. It was basically the grace of God, or something that just happened at the right time. It was just an accidental miracle."

Betty remembered, "I thought it was amazing. The realtor talked to Syd. Syd called Carolyn and said, 'I think this is it.' And he found it, like in July, after Jim died in May. It sure would have been nice for Jim to have seen this happen. But that's the way it worked."

Betty laughed when she said, "So when we found it we said, 'It needs a lot of work.' You could tell it had potential. But things just work out, because you couldn't have had a better set-up. The way the apartments connected was just perfect for what we needed at the time. People that we took over there said they liked Raymond's upstairs apartment better than the downstairs. Raymond's apartment had a warm cozy feeling to me, although Carolyn never did like the drapes in that living room. I think she hated them. The neighbor second door down donated them; they were plenty good for a guy's apartment.

As usual the family and some friends stepped in and started to work right away.

Betty remembered, "I think it was neat that Raymond was over there so much during renovation and was involved with everything. He spent a lot of days over there. We had the couch and the TV and remote all set up for him in the living room there on the first floor.

As Betty talked it was easy to picture Raymond on that couch in front of a TV with a Pepsi in his hand watching busy workers scraping and painting all round him.

"It was so surprising," Betty added, "The most work was on the first floor. It just amazed me how we worked and worked on the first floor, then Raymond went upstairs on the second floor and picked out his bedroom. I had wondered if he was going to pick out the first floor. It didn't work that way. Things just happen because they were meant to happen, you know?

"Oh my gosh, the back room where the previous owner slept must have leaked for years. So we had to put a whole new roof on. I got out there and rolled some tar paper. I wasn't as much help with that. We had to put new drywall up and plaster over that room. Then we had to take painted-over wallpaper off in the living room, dining room and the upstairs living room.

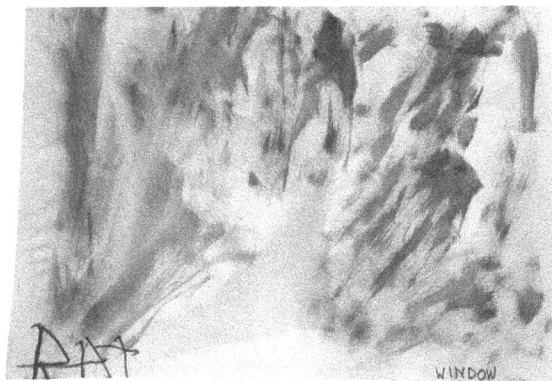

Raymond's painting "Window."

"The upstairs also had a dining room, and a kitchen. We closed that dining room off to make a second bedroom.

"Of course, at first the air conditioning was all window units. I couldn't believe that. There must have been six little air conditioners upstairs and downstairs. Syd just threw them all away. He put central air in and new hot water heaters. Of course Denise rewired it [Raymond's sister, an electrician, like her father].

"Syd can do anything and his family has any kind of tool you might need. It's nice if you have to do that kind of work to have the right equipment for it. He had a spiral notebook with a list of every thing that needed to be done and we'd go in each day and do every task and check them off.

"Carolyn, Denise, Millie, and I went over to strip wallpaper. Gerald helped. I learned of a tool with little points on it to run over the wall and spray water on it. It was hard work, but we got it all done."

Again this remarkable family pulled together and moved mountains to make life better for Raymond. Despite years of fear around Raymond moving away, both Raymond and the family made a smooth transition into his new home. Getting Raymond into the thick of remodeling and picking and choosing what would be done to his space may have given him a sense of control over what was going on for him. He no longer repeatedly expressed an earlier fear, "Don't move my stuff." He felt a positive connection to this building and to its transformation from the very beginning. When it was time for him to gradually take his things to the new house, he did it with pleasure and a sense of possession and hospitality. He even moved in unannounced when his already moved-in roommate Tony simply asked Raymond one evening during a visit if he'd like to go ahead and stay the night in his new room. Raymond said, "Yeah." And that was that.

Chapter 11

Recruitment

The group is busy discussing a persistent problem at a regular meeting.

"I don't understand why we haven't gotten any bites from students. That would be the ideal roommate; someone who is going to be home to study in the evenings, and give Raymond a hand, but will appreciate having free days for classes. And with two seminaries practically in walking distance from Raymond's house, you'd think people would be flocking in." Linda speculates about this as she chooses a delicious slice of pizza. "No mushrooms, no."

"We have had some luck with students, like Owen and Bryan." Nancy, a very strong recruiter, says this with a mixed positive and frustrated tone.

"We simply have to meet people and talk to them," Milton offers. "That is the only way to introduce them to being with Raymond. I remember sitting at this table interviewing people with Betty and Gerald. The people we were interviewing were probably thinking, 'What!' They were wondering who the boss would be. 'Who are all these people?'"

As Jo Ann suggested they do, the group is working on one particular issue at this meeting: recruitment. Raymond needs new support staff for his day, one or two or more people who will plan a good day with Raymond and spend that time regularly with him. Raymond also wants a roommate who will be there for his evenings and during the night.

"Hope's ads are great, and Gerald has updated them. We all need to put the flyers in places. So where are you putting ads, everybody!?" Carolyn wields her markers to begin a sort of map of likely ad placements.

"I'll put one over at Bellarmine University, and get Corie to put one at U of L, and I think I can get one in the Deer Park Newsletter. And I keep calling that guy at the Autism Training Center. I just never hear back from him," Julie puts in as she juggles pizza and a notebook.

"I'll have an ad at Springdale Presbyterian, and I've talked to some people there. I'll ask if I can get an ad in the *Southeast Christian Outlook*." Milton watches Carolyn add his items to the sheet on the wall.

"I don't understand why the churches don't have more interested people," Betty remarks. "I am going to talk to the pastors at Harvey Browne Presbyterian Church, and St. Matthew's Methodist, both right across the street here. There's a church on every corner in this part of town."

"Betty, we haven't gotten much response from churches, but neither have we had much from any other institution. I'll call the Presbyterian Center. They probably have a newsletter and communicate with all of the Presbyterian churches around town. Thank you," Nancy adds as Betty takes her paper plate and scoops a few other plates as she goes.

"Raymond, do you want any more pizza?"

"No." Raymond hands her his plate.

"Milton, you want another Pepsi?"

"No thank you, Raymond."

"Nancy?"

"No, I think I have had enough, Raymond. Thank you."

"Nancy, how's Birch?"

"Just fine. She tried to jump over the fence again yesterday, but I stopped that."

"No, don't anybody get up, there isn't room if we all start moving around. I've got them." Betty heads around to the little kitchen with her load of used paper plates.

Carolyn continues her flow chart of potential recruitment sources. Oprah quietly introduces another guest on the big screen in the corner, while Raymond watches intently. Oprah and her guests make the room feel even more crowded. Raymond doesn't mind.

"I am holding your feet to the fire," Carolyn threatens the group.

"Denise has run off a hundred more ad flyers, so we need to get them out and in people's hands," Betty says as she gets back into her chair just inside the door. "Gerald said he'd go on websites and use that as a way to recruit. I am going to ask him to get a copy of the ad, just the words, ready for Raymond's bulletin at Highland Pres."

Carolyn records that for Betty as Michelle offers, "I will take ads to the Baptist Seminary and to the Education Department at U of L."

The talk continues, and the ads do get delivered. But responses are slow and few. Raymond's part-time morning companion, Alex, is talking with one of his friends to see if he is interested in working with Raymond. He could work out as a roommate for Raymond. It is a lengthy process and a constant need; a persistent frustration for Raymond's circle.

Matching people with Raymond

Recruiting staff to assist in any person's day is a remarkably difficult task – essentially two jobs, maybe more. The first job is connecting with people to see who would like to work with Raymond. The second is persisting with that because of high turnover.

But there are a few people who work in human services, or are students interested in that field, or in pastoral work, or perhaps nursing, who might be interested in direct service work. There are people who are realizing that there is more room for people to work as what are being called "direct service professionals,"* or in some cases, "personal care attendants."* There are degree programs being developed at community colleges to train people to work as DSP's. There are support organizations developing around these workers. And there are people who just enjoy working closely with people. (Look these organizations up to learn more about this growing field: www.dswresourcescenter.org, www.nadsp.org, www.ancor.org, www.dspspeak.org.)

The task is to find these people, nudge them out of the woodwork, and see if they fit with someone like Raymond. Raymond's group tried every search avenue. Here are some:

1. Flyers placed on college and seminary and church job boards and community information boards.

2. PR brochures sent to neighborhood and community center newsletters, area newspapers, church bulletins.

3. E-networking, through e-mail and information-sharing bulletin boards on related websites.

4. Brochures and handshakes shared between friends; networking at community events, church socials, professional meetings, board meetings, town meetings, volunteer gatherings. Word-of-mouth contacts proved to be the best source of new recruits for Raymond.

Sales professionals say that it takes seven contacts before a sale is closed. The group would repeat sayings like that in order to stave off discouragement. Not every person recruited filled the bill just right. It was left to trial and error to see what worked for the worker, and for Raymond.

At one point in the constant effort to "close the sale," Milton presented a profile of "Raymond's Ideal Support Person." It was definitely "Ideal," but it gave the group a target to aim for:

RAYMOND'S IDEAL SUPPORT PERSON

Personal Skills and Characteristics

Initiative: restlessness with status quo, continually looking for way to improve/refine things for Raymond

Creativity: ability to get past barriers and visualize positive possibilities

Tenacity: not giving up when things don't work the first time

Self Motivation: ability to think on one's feet and function autonomously, without close supervision

Commitment: to Raymond and his family

Organizational Skills: ability to develop and plan well in advance – can organize time supporting Raymond – including time developing additional opportunities for Raymond and follow-up with folks where Raymond is spending "liberated time" (free of human service types)

Negotiation: ability to work with community people to figure out positive ways for Raymond to fit into all or a part of what it is that they do – including facilitating ways for Raymond to be involved in valued activities without any human service types hanging around

Dependability: "no surprises" – ability to follow through with things that are planned

Interpersonal Skills: has a professional yet personable manner, can meet the public, conveys a positive image of self and Raymond, can talk about issues using everyday language, and can build a sense of commonality (regarding self, Raymond, and other community members)

Knowledge of the Community: and/ or willingness to explore

Belief : that Raymond can and must have a valued place within his community

Compensation
Living Wage: something reasonably commensurate with the skills/characteristics needed – at least twice that of a fry cook at McDonalds

Desirable Background
Restless human services/education/public relations worker

College student (perhaps art or music major, to be creative)

Does not require formal human services education or training except (there are ways to learn about these after being hired if the person so desires):

Basics of instruction: including ways to plan instruction in new activities, appreciating the ways that such activities are typically learned, and ways to promote the involvement of typical community people in Raymond's learning about new things

Social role valorization theory*: including an appreciation of the need to know Raymond and the impact that groupings of people, places, and activities will have on Raymond's community involvement

Matching Raymond with people
Another task necessary to recruit and match a person to spend quality time with Raymond, or a person like Raymond, was to find out who Raymond would want to be with, and how he would want them to spend his day with him. Since Raymond was

not one to be overtly specific about what he liked in people, the group had to guess by what had been successful for Raymond and with whom he had gotten along.

The group spent some time developing a profile of Raymond to help introduce him to a prospective recruit. This draft sheet was circulated for everyone in the group to add to. It asked each person to summarize their awareness of things that affected Raymond strongly.

It began: "This is intended to be a simple introduction to Raymond and the ways that we as his friends have discovered to make our time with Raymond as comfortable and interesting as possible for him and for us. With this information, a new person meeting Raymond for the first time would benefit from our years of experience, and get to know Raymond with some of Raymond's' 'language' in place beforehand."

Nancy sent her draft back with lots of suggestions. Since she spent a lot of time with Raymond and his family, her input was especially valuable. Here are some of her replies:

Please list things you have found that make Raymond particularly uncomfortable.

1. Frustration at not being able to complete a task himself, e.g., coat sleeves that get messed up; not being able to get at his wallet

2. Other people getting upset, angry, or frustrated

3. Rooms that are too dark and/or noisy, particularly restaurants

4. People talking about things in front of him that make him uncomfortable, like describing new situations or those which were difficult for him

State some other examples of things that are hard for Raymond:

5. Surprises

6. New people around who have not been introduced

7. Touching new things, or being unexpectedly touched

8. New textures, materials, or unfamiliar foods

9. Loud or persistent sounds or music

10. Storms or major changes in weather

11. Small children who cry or act needy

Raymond could tolerate these things for short times if people explained why or how they were happening, and how they might affect him. Because, for whatever reason, Raymond didn't take in all that was around him in the ways most of us do, it was important for trusted people around him to give him information he wasn't getting other ways.

Please list things you have found that Raymond enjoys:

1. Stopping for a Pepsi, and picking up a paper for Betty

2. Buying presents and cards and surprises for others and presenting them

3. Spending time with his brother and sisters; looking briefly after Carolyn's kids

4. Being asked to help someone run errands

5. Keeping track of phone messages, and having brief phone conversations

6. Having visitors at home, while he can relax and do his own thing

7. Television at home

8. Hamburger places, fish sandwiches and pizza restaurants

9. Anticipation and preparation of fish frys

10. Picking up family at the airport

11. Visiting Meemaw

12. Going to art class

13. Spending time with people who genuinely like Raymond

An ideal day for Raymond would be:

Running errands; doing a job or volunteer work for a few hours; lunching with friends; spending the evening at Owen's; having visitors over; relaxing at home

What have you found to help Raymond be most at ease and productive?

1. Those around him being at ease and relaxed

2. Beforehand knowledge of what's on the agenda

3. Doing things with others that they are enthusiastic about

4. Trusting someone for support through the rough spots

5. Sincere thanks for work he has accomplished, assistance he has given

When people are different in their means and methods of connecting with others and with their world, it is necessary for a new person in their life to have a fresh view of how to meet and relate to them. But if we get away from the usual patterns of interaction that most people learn, we have more success connecting with someone like Raymond who is so direct and honest in his way of relating.

Raymond's friend Milton Tyree has a gift for relating to people this way. He intuitively peels away the rind of social habits and cuts to the real "yes" and "no" of how to listen and hear what a person is truly saying and doing. He sent a draft on relating to

Raymond that was unlike all the others. It provided deep insight into what getting along with Raymond, and other people who don't fit the round hole, could be like ideally.

"NO!"

According to Peter Block, "no" is the beginning of the conversation for change. "If I cannot say no, then my yes means nothing. The act of refusal is the beginning of a new conversation."

If Mr. Block is correct, then Raymond was the consummate conversation starter. Problem was, that "NO" was the beginning and the end – of almost everything. NO was known. NO was safe. NO was static. NO had taken on an immense impoverishing power – it was sucking the life out of Raymond, Betty, Jim, and anyone else who cared to take a genuine look. What about Raymond's choice in the matter? Doesn't he have the "right" to say "NO"? Sure. But CHOICE implies options. At first there were none for Raymond..

Captured in differentness, consumed by failure – liberation for Raymond meant discovery of the ordinary. Raymond needed to get out of the door. He needed to explore.

How could folks supporting Raymond orchestrate circumstances for new possibilities? What needed to be in place to create the likelihood for success?

These were some ideas that could be provided to support people to get started:

Do take the time to explain. Be truthful about plans. Much will hinge on the integrity of your relationship with Raymond (e.g., "I can't drive my car today because it needs new brakes." Or, "Today we need to go at 10:00 for your blood-work. I know it is difficult, but it's important. I'll go with you and things will be OK.").

Don't sugar coat, or assume that Raymond won't understand.

Do listen.

Don't try to talk away Raymond's anxiety or wishes. (This does not mean that you have to do everything Raymond wants to do. It means that you listen in a way that he feels his desires and concerns are heard.)

Do invite and gently encourage Raymond to do new things (e.g., "This looks like an interesting place to visit. Let's go to the new gym at Bellarmine and see what it is like." Or, "I need your help with this. Please set the number of copies to 5 and hit the start button.").

Don't make it easy for Raymond to stay in the dark, and end the discussion with "No" (e.g., "Do you want to go to the new gym?" "Do you want to make copies?"). Often, it is easier for Raymond to say no than risk failure.

Do provide ways that Raymond can contribute – enliven his innate desire to do things for others.

Don't *allow things to unfold in a way where Raymond continually finds himself on the receiving end of help. This will deaden his spirit.*

Do be "planful" and foster opportunities for success. For instance, invite Raymond to get involved in an activity by assisting you – because he likes to be helpful. Begin with parts that will go well for him; e.g., if making copies for the first time, begin by asking him to raise the cover and hit the copy button since neither of these require precise movements. Then gradually add steps of increasing difficulty including the positioning of paper, setting the machine for the number of copies to be made, etc., until he is doing as much as possible by himself.
Don't *just "show up" and set Raymond up for failure because of poor planning.*

Do plan for Raymond to learn to do some things by himself.
Don't *make him believe that he must always have someone help him.*

Do involve typical community people when Raymond is learning new things. Who is the person who typically welcomes new people, helps them learn the ropes, and so forth? In other words, be a bridge, or one who orchestrates things working well for Raymond and the new people he meets. Discern when to get involved and when to get out of the way.
Don't *take charge of making all of the decisions about Raymond's learning new things in the community – unless you want to convince others that they could never be involved with him without your "expertise" or "intervention."*

Do show Raymond that you have high expectations by presenting suitably challenging things for him to do and learn.
Don't *underestimate him.*

Do take Raymond seriously – treat him like an adult. The Golden Rule is helpful here.
Don't *trivialize Raymond's words, feelings, thoughts, or time.*

Do devote time to really know Raymond and appreciate all of the things that he has to contribute.
Don't *know him only by the things that are difficult for him to do.*

Do Celebrate Commonality – talk to others about Raymond's contributions and commonality. We need to move beyond the bumper sticker mentality of Celebrating Diversity and Tolerance. People realizing what they have in common with Raymond – appreciating their mutuality – will provide the spark for the genuine, reciprocal, balanced relationships he needs. Raymond doesn't need to be tolerated. He needs to be understood, known, and loved.
Don't *talk about Raymond as though he is a client, and emphasize the things he cannot do.*

Do be honest (with Raymond and others) about your relationship and role with

Raymond (e.g., "I'm someone who is helping Raymond make new connections with people and places in his community. He's interested in photography, and I want to get some ideas from you about ways he can learn more.").

Don't *misrepresent yourself or confuse relationship roles for Raymond or others.*

Do (from Herb Lovett) tell Raymond you think you understand what is happening when he's having a difficult time. Advise Raymond to "yell if you need to yell." Try to gently negotiate (as Owen has done): "Yell if you need to yell, but please don't bang on the walls." Such negotiation will work best when not in the heat of the moment.

Don't *tell Raymond to control himself when things are not going well. This will only worsen the situation. (Who else, when upset, calms down when asked to do so?)*

Do appreciate the complexity and mystery surrounding some of the ways that Raymond behaves, processes information. . . . The fact is, we don't always know why Raymond does the things he does, and neither does he: what's within his control, and what's not? (Sometimes we may know or have a good guess, but at other times everyone may be at a total loss.)

Don't *try to simplify everything to ABC (antecedent, behavior, consequence) behavioral theory.**

If we applied these same do's and don'ts to anyone/everyone, wouldn't this be a much more understanding and comfortable world to live in? Of course there are elements here that apply more to Raymond than to the rest of us, but think through Milton's words one more time using your name, or the name of a loved one, a child that you care about, a friend living with a disability, or even someone you fear – in place of Raymond's name. We might all spend that time and think about it. It could do us some good.

Chapter 12

Finding Funding

I magine that you needed someone to be with you nearly twenty-four hours a day. Whether for physical help, or for support in communication, or simply to structure your day in a way that made it possible for you to move out into the community, how would you pay that person that supports you?

People who are in charge of institutional care, such as nursing homes, convalescent care, and other medically-oriented facilities believe that the care they give warrants the high cost of providing that care. For a long time, institutions held a monopolistic grip on the government funds made available to provide such care. Creative alternatives to institutional care were difficult to initiate and support because of lack of funding and the weight of the "red tape" which protected the medical model* of institutional care.

In some circumstances, particularly for those with extremely fragile health or dementia, or no community support whatsoever, that type of medical facility may be appropriate and necessary.

People who have investigated the disparity between institutional costs and home-based care costs believe that "home is where the heart is." People who have studied the effects of environment on overall health know that being in familiar surroundings with people that you care about is much better than living with a whole lot of strangers confined together. Also living in an environment that you have choices about, where the things in that space are yours and you can move and dispose them in the ways that you want, is less stressful and thus mentally and physically healthier.

Luckily, the trend has been, in the past fifteen years especially, toward promoting community integration of people living with disability, as opposed to institutional living. However this idea of community integration takes several forms and some of these forms are devolving back into the direction of institutional-type care.

Many people see the situation Raymond eventually had as close to ideal. He was living in his own home, making choices about how it looked and who lived there with him. This made Raymond comfortable and pleased with his situation.

The fine line between institution and community integration

The community integration most people with disabilities experience is less autonomous than Raymond's situation and often less integrated. Instead of the multi-bed institution, people live in group homes, staffed residences, apartments, or congregate living, or with family home providers. First, these are the programs that the Community Based Waivers* of Medicaid usually support, so they are the programs that most people are participating in.

The Medicaid Community-Based Attendant Services and Supports Act of 2003 amended title XIX (Medicaid) of the Social Security Act (SSA) to allow what became known at the Medicaid Waivers. This made possible the coverage of community-based attendant services and supports for certain Medicaid-eligible individuals.

Medicaid was initially – and is still chiefly – geared to funding institutions and long term care facilities; but the Community Based Waivers give nod to the increased desire of people to live in homes out in the community rather than in nursing facilities and state hospitals.

States may offer a variety of services to consumers under an HCBS* (Home and Community Based Services) waiver program and the number of services that can be provided is set by each state's legislature, and service prerogatives.

> These programs may provide a combination of both traditional medical services (i.e. dental services, skilled nursing services) as well as non-medical services (i.e. respite, case management, environmental modifications). Family members and friends may be providers of waiver services if they meet the specified provider qualifications. However, in general spouses and parents of minor children cannot be paid providers of waiver services.... The HCBS waiver program in particular is a viable option for states to use to provide integrated community-based long-term care services and supports to qualified Medicaid eligible recipients.
> (www.cms.hhs.gov/MedicaidStWaivProgDemoPGI/)

With the HCBS waiver, states have the option to build flexible programs that best serve the people in those states, provided the administrators show:

1. That their waiver services will on the whole cost less than an institution providing similar services.

2. That the health and welfare of their consumers will be protected.

3. That there will be sufficient and reasonable providers available to meet the needs of the people involved.

4. That providers develop and provide services in accord with a plan of care.

Most people who receive Supplemental Security Income (SSI) are Medicaid recipients; consequently, in Kentucky, if they are considered mentally retarded and developmentally disabled and would be at risk of living in an institution without this funding, they can apply for Supports for Community Living, one of Kentucky's four 1915C Medicaid waiver programs, in order to live outside of an institution.

As Mary Johnson of the Advocado Press says, "Why is this still a waiver? Why is it not the normative funding?" Expedience? Group homes can house anywhere from three to eight residents, depending on local ordinances. You can hire fewer staff to care for more individuals than in a person's own home. Staffed residences can also have more people living together with varying needs, and thus require less direct-care staff. Family home providers often make a home into a comfortable place for a person or three to live, but it is still the home of the provider, not the resident.

Advocates in the disability rights movement have been working for years to support people's hopes of living in places of their choice that compare to living in any general community. Since even before the Americans With Disabilities Act (ADA)* was passed in 1990, which mandated equal access in the marketplace for people living with disabilities, advocates have been working toward making it simple for people to live in their own homes with the personal care and financial support to make that possible.

In 1998, "The Medicaid Community Attendant Services and Supports Act, designed to reform the Medicaid program by allowing people a choice to remain at home rather than go to a nursing home, was introduced in the Senate by Sen. Tom Harkin (D-IA) and co-sponsored by Senator Arlen Specter (R-PA) . . . " ("MiCassa", *Ragged Edge,* Advocado Press) www.raggededgemagazine.com/focus/micassa0804.html

"In 1998 Medicaid spent $44 billion in reimbursements to institutions, according to figures from the Health Care Financing Administration*, but only $14 billion on home and community-based services, or just 25% of its total long-term care expenditures. According to data gathered by the University of California/San Francisco's Disability Statistics Center, the average yearly Medicaid expenditure for a person using community-based services was $7,276, compared to a taxpayer cost of $23,225 for a person receiving Medicaid services in a nursing home [mid- 90s figures]."

Such differences in costs were beginning to be noted by people concerned with disability issues, and legislation continued to be sponsored to make living at home a better option than institutionalization for people receiving Medicaid funds.

In 2004 1915c HCBS waiver expenditures per person in the U.S. totaled $20,197. In Kentucky the average total expenditure for a person was $12,455. In 2005 in the U.S. 43% of Medicaid funding was spent on care for people in nursing facilities, while 40.9 % was spent on home-based services. In Kentucky 55.6% was spent on institutional care while 31.5% was spent on home-based services. http://www.statehealthfacts.org/comparetable

It needs to be noted that the figure of $20,197 above represents average costs for services for a person who needs basic part-time home care, and administers their own funding. It would not cover services for a person who needs support coordination*, day habilitation*, residential support, or paid roommates or wrap-around support* staff. These services push a person's financial needs closer to those of a person living in a nursing facility. These combined services in 2008 can cost upwards of $50,000 annually. To compare, private pay for a nursing facility "bed" cost $70,000+ per year in 2006. (Sept. 11 2006, Senior Journal.com)

Current legislative efforts are refining the methods of delivering funding to people with disabilities for appropriate care services. States are supporting pilot programs of Consumer Directed Options for funds distribution (see also Chapter 14). The Community Choice Act* is under consideration by Congress in 2008.

Coordinating funding sources

There is no way around it; living out in the community and needing a high level of care and supervision is still expensive, although it is believed to be less so than institutional care. The trick to funding community care is intensive researching of what funds exist and finding out how they could be made available to the person you are caring for.

Connecting with agencies

A key to accessing this constellation of funding sources is close communication with providers in your community who are offering the services that are paid for by those funds' sources. And it is a good idea to put people on your team who are veterans of the funding wars. Everyone who has cared for someone with developmental disabilities in your community has had to wade into the morass of programs that offer different pots of money for different things and situations that a dependent person needs. These funds are administered by state government bureaucracies, or by comprehensive care agencies. Such agencies (like Seven Counties, mentioned as a support for Raymond) are usually board-directed non-profit agencies mandated by government bureaucracies and beholden to them for their structure and for pass-through funds. Dealing with the complexity of these agencies can seem to be deep, convoluted, and almost impossible to navigate. But with savvy agency personnel as group contacts, much can be accomplished.

You might recall scenes in the wonderful classic film *The African Queen,* with Katherine Hepburn and Humphrey Bogart, when you think of such "navigation." If you have seen it, you might remember when Rosie the missionary and Charlie the river-rat are escaping the German army. Exhausted from navigating rough river rapids, they fall asleep in his boat as it floats into the trackless channels of an African river delta. When they wake they are partly aground surrounded by a dense swamp of tall matted grasses in shoulder-deep water. They have to drag the boat through endless passages of this murky, leech-infested, mosquito-swarming horror with little hope of ever finding the open river again. They don't know where they are going, and they have no idea how to get there, and while they are struggling to keep going the journey is dreadful and arduous. But don't lose hope. Rosie and Charlie didn't, and they did find a way out, and joyously got out onto the open lake and, oops, then were captured by the German Navy. Oh, well.

So it could be said, "Oh, heavens, don't even try." Better would be, "Don't go it alone, whatever you do. Befriend experts!"

As Tim said about Raymond's group, "Raymond had a group of people who were dedicated to fighting against that nonsense [bureaucratic obfuscation] and bringing some kind of semblance of order out of the chaos.

"It is not that the system isn't functioning for people but I don't think there is the impetus unless there are individuals going to the system and saying let's make this happen, Let us make this work for this person."

Again, the key is what works for the individual.

Tim continued, "Yet I think that exactly the opposite is sometimes true, that the system is functioning against people. I am personally of the opinion that there is invidious intent underneath."

Tim's years working within the system made it hard for him to believe that there wasn't an underlying motivation built into the "system" to make it hard for people to access needed benefits and services. And maybe he was right. That makes it that much more important for people to act together on behalf of people who can't advocate for themselves.

Cindy Bayes concurred with Tim's opinion but felt that the difference in Raymond's group was that people "in the system" were working to make it work for Raymond. (For example, Cindy is Seven Counties' Division Director /Specialized Services.)

"That's really right," she agreed. "Whether it was Seven Counties or Community Employment or others, the agencies knew that colleagues were involved and that Raymond's group had a reputation and longevity and were going to be watching. I don't know if it was all about that watching or the accountability that made it stand out."

Cindy was considering this carefully, since it could make a difference for others trying to make the "system" work. "I think it was a couple of things. One of them was the group's independence. You, as a group, could dance over and ask the system something and if you didn't like what they said you danced away. Likewise we in the system would dance over and say, 'What can we do?' or answer your questions.

"Sometimes what you asked didn't fit into the services boxes or into the AIS slot or those sorts of things. Sometimes I wish the dance could have worked better. But I think some of your success was the strength of your 'intimidation.' There was your strong will to get things done that the service system didn't always understand. And you didn't always understand what the service system what trying to do. We always needed to work better together."

Despite Cindy's doubts about all of that action, the two visiting camps worked pretty well over the years.

Raymond's primary funding sources were:

SSI – Supplemental Security Income, allowing him to be eligible for Medicaid, and thus the Supports for Community Living Waiver.

SSDI – Social Security Disability Income, drawn on his parents' accounts and making him eligible for Medicare.

Supported Living – Passed in Kentucky in 1992, a statute which offers to fund a number of flexible individualized services designed to provide the necessary assistance to enable a person to live in a home of choice, participate in the community, have rights and autonomy promoted, enhance one's skills and competency to live in the community, and promote community acceptance through home ownership or leasing. Supported Living does not fund services which Supports for Community Living covers. The funds are accessed by grant application, and a limited number of grants are awarded each year.

Carolyn Wheeler was one of the forces behind making Supported Living a way to fill the gaps that funding from the Supports for Community Living Waiver would necessarily have. Here she shares her experience of the beginning of Supported Living:

> I can still recall sitting beside Jane Hart at a conference . . . in the spring of 1991. Jane, as always, was involved in her usual "doodle art" while listening to the speaker talk about such wonderful things as people with disabilities planning and living, to a greater extent than I had ever thought possible, lives that reflected their personal interests and choices. The paradigm shift from group home to real home, programs to supports, and client-hood to citizen had yet to be birthed in Kentucky.

> Jane and I began whispering (yes, this was rude as the speaker was still talking) about who we could bring together to think about a new way of providing services in Kentucky. Since November of 1990, I had been involved with what was for me a new way of thinking about and planning for people with significant disabilities. Through a federal grant, I was facilitating a number of Personal Futures Planning teams for young adults with deaf /blindness as part of the transition planning process from high school. Since the typical transition outcome for many of these young adults was to graduate and just be at home without any kind of meaningful work or post-secondary option, we were hopeful we could achieve a greater degree of success in creating a richer life for both the student and his/her family.

> Based on the same process that was involved in Raymond's circle, we were

finding these teams could develop images of the future which actually were what most people would just consider a "normal" life – having a place of one's own, a job that paid a decent wage, going on vacation, being a member of a faith community or organization with shared interests, having friends, getting a driver's license – basically the "American Dream." However, without public resources to pay for people to provide the needed support, these dreams would just remain as nice ideas and images on easel paper.

So, on that little pad of paper they give you at these conferences with the hotel's name and address, Jane and I made a list of people to invite to talk about the lack of resources in Kentucky to help people with disabilities to live ordinary lives in their communities. Jane hosted a gathering at the Frankfort County Club, and Hope Leet Dittmeier graciously agreed to facilitate the meeting. Out of that day-long meeting developed a smaller group of people who agreed to learn about a relatively new concept being developed in other states called Supported Living.

Somehow, (although I personally don't believe in coincidences but in Providence), a copy of Gary Smith's book on the topic of Supported Living had arrived in my mailbox at work. As a publication of the National Association of State Mental Retardation/Developmental Disabilities Program Directors, this book became the foundation for this effort. (Gary Smith, *Supported Living: New Directions in Services for People with Developmental Disabilities,* Alexandria, VA: National Association of State Directors of Developmental Disabilities Services, 1990.) Copies were ordered and distributed to our Task Force. This became the basis of our learning – we read about the states' programs which were identified as having promise, and four of us visited programs in Ohio and Illinois. We got copies of their legislation and began learning about how this worked. Jane arranged for testimony before the Joint House/Senate Committees on Health and Welfare of our General Assembly where parents and people with disabilities were able to share their dreams for their future and their frustration and actual despair in having no hope this would ever be realized.

An unexpected champion for this effort emerged from this public hearing. Bob Heleringer, who at that time was a State Representative (in the Kentucky State Legislature) from Louisville, agreed to sponsor legislation for a Supported Living program. Rep. Heleringer was an unexpected ally as he was a long-term advocate and supporter of institutional services for folks with mental retardation and developmental disabilities. However, he also saw and supported the need for expansion in community services and resources. His assistance with the Legislative Research Commission in this process was invaluable to the end result. Our little group continued to meet with him and also had the opportunity to revise the legislation. On March 17, 1992, the legislation was passed and Supported Living was "birthed" in Kentucky.

The design of Kentucky's Supported Living program was quite unique in that people had to make application for the funding. This required the completion of an application and a budget request. (See page 92 for the letter accompanying Betty's application.) This was really the beginning of what is now referred to as "self-directed supports" and "individual budgets" and is gaining wide acceptance and implementation in many Medicaid waiver programs throughout the United States. Because several of the key Supported Living advocates were also members of Raymond's circle, an application to Supported Living was made in the fall of 1992.

Betty applied for Supported Living funds in November 1992, only nine months after the program was presented as a Bill (HB No. 447 General Assembly, Commonwealth of Kentucky) to the Kentucky Legislature. The program was called Supported Living for these reasons stated in the Bill:

(5) "Supported Living" means a broad category of highly flexible, individualized services designed and coordinated in such a manner as to provide the necessary assistance to do the following:

a. Provide the support necessary to enable a person who is disabled to live in a home of the person's choice which is typical of those living arrangements in which persons without disabilities reside;

b. Encourage the individual's integrated participation in the community with persons who are members of the general citizenry;

c. Promote the individual's rights and autonomy;

d. Enhance the individual's skills and competences in living in the community; and

e. Enable the individual's acceptance in the community by promoting home ownership or leasing arrangements in the name of the individual or the individual's family or guardian.

To distinguish the funding offered by Supported Living from that often available through the Community Based Waiver (in Kentucky, Supports For Community Living, Home and Community Based Waiver, and Traumatic Brain Injury Assistance) the Bill excluded "the following housing arrangements:

a. Segregated living models such as any housing situation which physically or socially isolates people with disabilities from general citizens of the community;

b. Congregate living models such as any housing situation which groups individuals with disabilities as an enclave within an integrated setting;

c. Any model where the individual, as an adult, does not have maximum control of the home environment commensurate with the individual's disabilities; and

   d. Any single living unit where more than three (3) people with disabilities live."

The emphasis, of course, is on supporting the more autonomous living arrangements for individuals.

Betty was encouraged to apply because the funding would work for Raymond while he still lived in his family home. At the time she applied, the circle's dream of Raymond's own home was still just a picture on a sheet of paper on the wall.

Here is Betty's application letter for Supported Living from November 19, 1992:

To Whom It May Concern,

I am writing this letter to ask for continued support of funding for my son Raymond. He is currently involved with the Passports/Outreach programs, but this funding will expire in June of 1993. The current funds allotted for Raymond in these programs is not adequate to meet his needs as outlined on his application.

Until Raymond's involvement with these programs, and having a Personal Futures Planning group, Raymond was totally depressed and house/couch bound. With Raymond's aggressive behavior, the entire family was at wits' end trying to find help and resources. I have found by Raymond getting involved in the community resource development program, and getting involved with real community life, he has made much progress in how he deals with people. You can most certainly tell by his actions, he feels better about himself. This has given our family a great deal of relief and hope.

I fear we may lose what has been accomplished thus far on Raymond's and our family's behalf unless I can find additional funding for Raymond's programs. When Raymond's programs lose funding, Raymond's life will be GREATLY diminished, as will our entire family's. My deepest fear is that the unity of the family will be at dire risk!

The consultation efforts, as requested, will focus on continuing Raymond's Personal Futures Planning group and coordinating efforts of those working on Raymond's behalf. I know that the amount of community resource funds I am requesting is more than Raymond is receiving now, but it will give the consultant funds to activate such activities as the Personal Futures Planning group deems appropriate for Raymond's future needs.

I appreciate you taking a moment to read this letter and the time you have spent in reviewing Raymond's application. If you have any questions at all, please feel free to call me at any time at . . .

Betty was requesting $250 a week to pay for a community resource developer, who provided a part-time (twenty hours per week) day support for Raymond, and a community living consultant who worked directly with Betty to coordinate any supports that she needed to keep Raymond successful in his home situation. Each year, the group would look at Raymond's situation and decide what would continue to need funding, and for what new efforts support should be requested. Each year Betty, often with help from Milton, Nancy, and Hope would compose the necessary application materials and letters of support.

Here is a copy of the letter that Betty and Milton wrote to request continued Supported Living funds for fiscal year 2000. There is a big difference from eight years before:

Dear Council Members:

In September 1991 Raymond would not leave the house. Nor did he want me to leave the house. His behavior was outrageous He was the most unhappy person I'd want to meet.

Then I met Jo Ann Boyle at a workshop about behavior problems. She worked at REACH and offered to convene a group of people including family, friends, and service providers to envision a positive future for Raymond. While I was unsure of what good may come of this, I was willing to try.

In 1991 I was trying to envision Raymond getting off of the couch. I would not have believed that eight years later he would be living in his own place and working.

Members of the group believed in Raymond, and they were instrumental in thinking about him having a life. Months later he was willing to leave the house, and the group started looking for community connections. Now the problem was not a lack of things Raymond was willing to do. It was a lack of resources to make things happen.

In 1993 Supported Living provided the resources to move ahead. Raymond's world grew. He was going out of town (instead of just off the couch earlier in the year), joining a gym, becoming a member of his community. His posture was different. Everyone could tell the change.

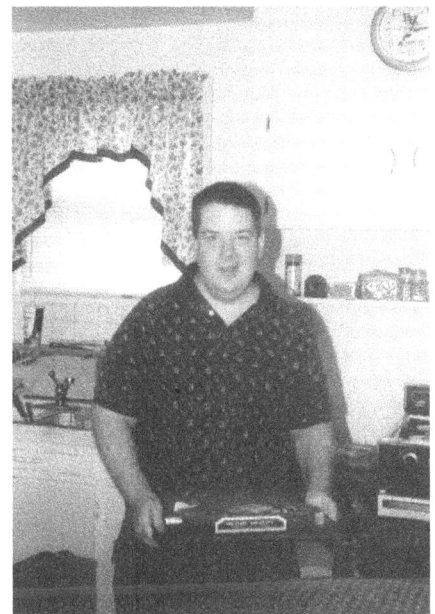

Raymond cooking in his apartment.

There have been ups and down. Difficult behaviors have resurfaced. There have been problems recruiting, training, and keeping suitable people to support Raymond. But, the group (which has stayed together since 1991), Raymond's family, and Supported Living, have remained steadfast.

In June 1999 Raymond moved to his own apartment. It's the biggest step that Raymond and I have ever taken. He stepped up to the plate. To me, it was amazing! Additional resources from Supported Living made this dream a reality.

Of course his transition is still in progress as Raymond learns more about the roles of roommate and neighbor. And I like the sound of "roommate' and "neighbor." Nine years ago, this would not have seemed possible.

I want to thank the Regional Supported Living Council for their support and flexibility through the years. Raymond did not need a program. (Unfortunately he'd been dismissed from many.) Raymond needed Supported Living. His life and mine have been as different as daylight and dark.

Our budget for this year ($37,716) reflects a $7,716 decrease of the current budget of $45,432. We no longer need the Family Broker since Lee Bobzien, SCS Case Manager, is covering these responsibilities. Also deleted was Community Resource Developer because the Day Habilitation person, paid through the Supports for Community Living Waiver, is supported by a sub-committee from Raymond's group in performing these functions. Emergency response is no longer needed as Raymond has become established in his own home. Art therapy and the one-time expense for home furnishings represent other savings.

One area of focus for Raymond's group is the efficient use and coordination of his supports for home and community. For instance, Raymond gets Section 8 support for housing and a reduced phone rate. Community Employment provides work supports. Raymond gets other support during the day through the Supports for Community Living Waiver (day habilitation and respite). We have made every effort to avoid duplication of services. For example Raymond's supported living plan for his home has been rejected (in writing) by every available Medicaid vendor.

Raymond's group includes, and has included, many people substantially involved in Kentucky's Supported Living initiative as well as the Supports for Community Living Waiver, and other community services. (Including Hope Dittmeier, Carolyn Wheeler, Milton Tyree, Nancy Brucchieri, Linda McAuliffe, Lee Bobzien, and others.) I rely a great deal on their experience and guidance concerning services which will support Raymond in having a good life.

Thank you again for providing extraordinary opportunities for my extraordinary son. I will be glad to meet with the Council to provide more information and/or answer any questions.

Raymond's life takes all of the pieces: his family, the group, and Supported Living. Frankly without all of these pieces, life for him would be an existence, not a life.

Sincerely,
Betty Atherton

Betty requested funds to the above amount to cover a number of services: residential transition trainer; a roommate; a facilitator for the planning team; accounting help; Workers' Compensation for in-home staff; matching funds to pay necessary employment taxes; and a small amount of funds to support ongoing recruiting of support staff.

At this time, Linda McAuliffe, one of Raymond's group members, was serving as Area Administrator for Supports for Community Living, the Medicaid Waiver in Kentucky. She knew that Raymond's situation was likely not going to work under standard SCL funding.

In a letter of support to the Supported Living Council, Linda backed up the reason that Raymond especially needed Supported Living funds to allow him to live out on his own.

"Since Raymond became a co-recipient of both Supports for Community Living and Supported Living funds many years ago, there has naturally been a question of whether the funds have been duplicative in the residential area. Currently Raymond receives funding for his residential support arrangement through Supported Living."

Linda shows the difference here between what Supports for Community Living (Medicaid Waiver) can pay for, and what the state administered fund, Supported Living will cover.

"The SCL waiver is designed to provide residential support through family home providers or staffed residences. While many family home provider arrangements support only one SCL recipient, staffed residences usually have three people living in them. The level of funding typically does not allow agencies to provide support for less than three individuals.

"In addition, SCL does not fund residential arrangements for individuals that own or lease their own home. The lease or ownership must be in the agency's name.

"It is important to Raymond that he has his own apartment, since this offers him a sense of stability and security. Another factor in this situation is that none of the residential providers in this area are willing and able to provide the specialized residential support that Raymond needs and wants.

"In conclusion, it is my belief that the use of Supported Living funds to support Raymond's residential arrangement is appropriate. The current SCL waiver and the current local providers cannot support Raymond in the living situation he wants and needs."

Several members of Raymond's group had considerable know-how when it came to finding, targeting, and implementing resources to make his living situation the best it could be. Despite that there was persistence and hard work still necessary to keep the funding available each year. Betty saw to the follow-up of every penny spent, and with committee help and Carolyn's accounting assistance they kept careful records and reports. This care and tenacity also made it possible for Raymond to have the life that his family wanted for him.

An Unpleasant Intermezzo

Anytime a person receives any funding from government sources they, or the people who care for them, must keep a close eye on everything that transpires around those funds. Meticulous records must be kept on every penny that comes in and goes out. All bank statements must be retained and accounts kept precisely balanced to the penny. All records of money spent and all receipts are to be kept as documents to prove appropriate use of funds. Betty knew this and she and Carolyn kept meticulous records for everything that happened on Raymond's behalf.

Reports are required annually by each funding source, and by the court if there is adjudicated dependent status or needed guardianship for the person in your care. Records kept like this are key in any question that any agency may have about whether the person is still entitled to these funds. Somehow, despite the fact that a person may have been born with a disability and has shown no change in that condition since birth, the funding agencies will periodically question that disability and require that the disabled person go through an extensive series of tests, considerable questioning and investigation of their status as disabled, and reviews of any documentation pertaining to their care and maintenance. Be ready; be very, very ready.

Here is an example of what can occur, at any time, without warning. This account is from one group member who is guardian and SSI payee for a friend with autism and cognitive impairment.

A Season In Brazil

Before you get a mental picture of the Carnival, with swaying paraders in outrageous colorful feathered and jeweled but otherwise scanty costumes, and tall and tan and young and lovely girls from Ipanema walking down sunny wave-kissed beaches, consider a different Brazil. The cult movie by ex- "Python" Terry Gilliam is the *Brazil* I am referring to. It is a stunning declamation of the world of bureaucracy and how it dehumanizes.

If you have any contact with anyone who is a recipient of any kind of government funds, ask them what it is like dealing with the system before you take your first plunge. Don't jump into the Social Security ocean without instructions and really good scuba gear. If you need to be payee for a friend or family member, be sure to talk to others who have experienced working with SSI or Social Security so you will know how to prepare reports, to document everything that you do regarding any use of the funds, and to carefully read and question any information you receive about your funds or your friend's or family member's account.

Here is a little example of SSI Brazil. When you receive SSI payments (Supplemental Security Income, for people with disabilities who are unable to work full-time and need Medicaid health insurance), it is necessary for you or your payee to make at least one annual report. This consists of listing all of your income for the year; who decided how it would be spent; what was used for food and housing; what was used for personal expenses; and what was left over, if anything, at the end of the year. (And woe betide if you go over their regularly changeable limit on what you can hold in an account, because they have been known to come and take away all of your money for another whole year after that if you went over by even a few dollars.) You also need to let them know if you had any felony convictions in the past year, and where and with whom you or your friend is living. They also want to know what type of bank account you keep the funds in, and if you have any other accounts as well. Oh, and if you are payee for a dependent child, you must have proof that the child is getting medical treatment for any disabling condition he/she might have. In the not-so-fine print you are also told that any information that you give can be shared with anyone they want to share it with. "The law allows us to do this even if you do not agree to it." Yes, that is a direct quote from the SSI annual report form.

So heads up, everybody! Brazil 101, Class One, is over.

Class Two: After you have filled out the annual report form, the Social Security people put it in their "reading-the-forms" machine. Your form may get kicked out for not having exactly what the form reader wants to read on it. (They actually have different levels of reader for easy-to-read forms where not much changes from year to year to more complex readers for people with more money problems, I guess.) This will generate a new flurry of activity. Then around November, out of the blue, you may get a letter saying that you need to bring in all the bank statements you have back a year or three, and any other account information you might or might not be aware of, and your grandmother's maiden name and the names of the seven dwarves and Santa's reindeer; well, you get the picture. So you gather all this material from your meticulously-kept files, and you head down to the Social Security office, because you know as well as I do that hell will be frozen solid before caller one ever gets through the Social Security phone line.

You get into the building and you stand in the check-in line for a while. The lady tells you to take a seat and someone will be with you. You wait an hour or so and get called in to talk to a nice lady in a row of identical cubicles that seems a mile long. People are walking up and down the rows of cubicles poking into file cabinets just lining the outside edges of the cubicles. You pull out the many bank statements, and all of the checks still taped to the sheets of recycled paper that you use so you can copy them for the court's bi-annual report. You pull out any other information you have on banks around town, and their habits and policies, and of course the dwarves and the reindeer. The lady smiles and takes it all and makes copies and runs up and down and pokes in file cabinets and comes back to the desk and puts things into the computer. Then she says, "Well, I believe it is all in order." And if you don't get her name and extension number then, you are a fool. End of Class Two, Brazil 101.

Class Three starts with a letter that comes in December stating, in no uncertain terms, that your SSI for the next year has been cancelled and you have no recourse except to hire a team of crack lawyers and start the appeals process and if you don't do that within the next twenty-four hours, then, nah-nah-nah-nah-naaah-nah!! (At least, they didn't come in through your roof and shoot down your family, like in the movie *Brazil*, when a typing error caused the whole murderous situation.)

No, there is no explanation in the letter at all why this has happened. You first think about what it is like to live on the street (or for the friend you receive funds for to live on the street) and how good an insulator cardboard really is. Not funny? Not meant to be. This happens to people, often.

Class Four: What do you do to deal with this? Well, you don't take it sitting down. You start a ruckus. You cancel everything you planned for the next day, if you are able to take a personal day away from work, and you pull out every possible bit of information from the files that might in some way pertain to the SSI issue, including all of the forms that the previous lady copied. You pack it in order, and then you get a substantial snack together, and a good book, a crossword puzzle or two and a good pencil, and you put on a raincoat and get lots of quarters, lots, for parking and moving the car around. Then you head downtown to the Social Security office to spend the day in Brazil. You sign in and tell the lady in the intake window as much as you can without becoming "postal." Luckily for her they have those heavy acrylic bars screwed onto the wall outside her cubicle window. Then you find a cozy chair (good luck; most Social Security offices have rows and rows of hard chairs that make airplanes look like luxury suites, and they are usually all full.) and get out your knitting, or the good book. It is also fun to foment a little rebellion occasionally by announcing how long you've been waiting to new neighbors, because plenty of people will be called up before you are, and lots of them will have gotten there long after you. Three or four hours later (well, of course you ask at the window every hour on the hour, how much longer, please? and, "I have to feed my meter a few blocks away; would you please let them know I'll be back if they call me?"), you are called in and the nice man takes you to his cubicle. You pull out all your records and all the dates, and all the material you had been told to bring in for the previous meeting and you ask him point blank what on earth this is about.

He sits and reads your material, and he looks in his computer, and he reads your material and he asks a question or two, and then he wanders up and down the aisles a while looking in the file cabinets.

"Well, your file is not here. Yes, I do have it in the machine, and it does say that you were here on November 15th."

"Yes, I know I was," you want to say, "but why am I here today?" After some more rooting in cabinets and clicking on the machine the man says that the lady who you visited with in November probably didn't bother to close the information she had gotten, so it didn't get into the system, so the system assumed it was never there. "Oh, it shows here that you came on the 15th and that entries were made about what she had asked you to bring. She just didn't close it, so it did not go in to the appropriate memory." (The samba rhythms of Brazil ring in your head quietly) Then you ask if that means that she was in error, and that you or your friend will be getting the SSI after all. He says probably. And you say, "That ain't good enough. I want it in writing and I want your signature on it!" And he says, "I can't do that." So you say, "Then how can I know that my friend is going to get her payments this year?"

He then says that he will call you and send you a statement of benefits on the morrow. So you say, "Please give me your name and your extension number." And amazingly he does, but you won't know until you try it if it actually is his. You tell him if you don't get that account statement in two days he isn't hearing the last of you, as you smile and shake his hand and prepare to leave. In two days you receive phone confirmation of your friend's SSI benefits for the year to come.

In March a letter comes in the mail.

"It is mandatory that your friend and you, the payee, appear at a meeting scheduled for (three days later) with these records available."

It is so hard to believe that they still haven't got it straight. You know that it could take two weeks to arrange everyone's schedule to get them all together for a meeting in three days. You grab your trusty date book and immediately call the number of the man that you spoke with in November who seemed to have everything worked out.

You explain to him that you have received yet another letter about this same situation and a mandatory date to be at the Social Security office, which you know you cannot keep. He says that it is not his case, not on his records, and you say, "What does it take to make it your case?"

You tell him that you don't even know what the problem is. He kindly takes the time to look up the file and realizes that the problem is still the record of an irrevocable funeral account that was opened on your friend's behalf twenty years before. The account is reported every year to Social Security by bank account number and total accumulation in the untouchable fund.

"What do I need to do to prove to Social Security that this is the same account I have been reporting to you for twenty years?"

You take another morning off. You go to the branch bank which holds the trust. They tell you that you must go to their main office downtown. You raid the piggy bank for more quarters and head down. After a fifteen-minute parking search you jump out of the car and trot the two blocks to the bank.

The bank officer in the trust department is a little baffled by your request, but calls the funeral home, gets a faxed affidavit of the records of the trust. The bank adds their letter and notary seal concerning the trust, and an itemized statement of interest accumulation for the past five years. This is all put on bank letterhead in a bank envelope and you trot back to the car, and zip over a few more blocks, and into the security maze in the Social Security building. You are thinking of renting a room there, you quip to the guard. He doesn't look amused and you duck down the hall.

"I need to see Mr. J. I have material that he requested yesterday." You know that he is here because you saw him duck his head out the door and call a name for another interview.

"Do you have an appointment?"

"I simply need to put these in his hands, that is all. And I need to do it now."

"I'll see what I can do," the lady smiles, "Please take a seat."

In a surprisingly short time (twenty minutes) your name is called. Another man's head is sticking out the door. You follow him into the maze.

"Do you have an appointment?" he asks redundantly.

"I simply need to put these papers into Mr. J's hands."

"Well, I am sorry, he is in an interview, what can I do for you?"

As he says this, you spot Mr. J heading down the corridor toward you and the file cabinet near you. You whip up out of your chair and politely block Mr. J's way and offer him the stack of papers that you garnered from the funeral home and bank. He graciously takes them, and you say, "Will you be needing anymore documentation on this account?"

"I'll let you know."

You briskly thank the other man who was sent to further obfuscate the situation and you leave, heading back through the maze till you find the door. All you can do now is wait for the next demand from these people, in your constant quest to protect your friend's minimal annual income from being revoked.

I noticed a small article in the back of the Sunday paper April 16, 2006, that said Medicaid will soon be requiring an individual to show a birth certificate or passport to be eligible for their Medicaid funding. Let's think about this: How many people who are on Medicaid are really able to apply for a birth certificate or a passport? How many would have seen that article? How many will get a letter next year demanding that they be in the SSI office the next day because of discrepancies in their records regarding their birth certificates?

I have since spent 10 months trying to trace records of my friend's birth. After a court appearance and trips to two local hospitals, several certified letters sent and months of phone calls, I found her birth certificate under a different birth name. Another friend, a refugee from war in Africa, recently asked me to read to her the letter saying she would need to present a birth certificate for her children to receive Medicaid. Now where will she get birth certificates for herself and her kids?

Lesson, and review: In *Brazil*, the movie, you are at fault until proven innocent. It is like France. So because the first lady didn't do the requisite final click, you, or your friend could have lost an annual income. Your income for her click. Mind you, it is no income to write home about, but it is your friend's annual income. How many people who are regular recipients of SSI, like Raymond, would have a clue what to do if they got arbitrarily cancelled like that? And that is only the beginning. Deal with this every year or so for twenty, thirty years, like Betty, and see if you don't break out in hives whenever there is an envelope marked "Social Security Administration" in your mailbox.

Chapter 13

Working – Making a Day for Raymond

Having a meaningful day? What does that involve for you? Take just a minute and write on your notepad or the back of that bank receipt just what makes a day meaningful for you, you only.

Done? Good. What made your day meaningful? Was it time with friends and family? Time to do something you feel is productive? Did you want solitary time, for work or gardening or hobby? Did you include time for physical labor or exercise or sports with your team or riding with the bike club? Do you need time for prayer, or time for play and entertainment?

Everyone finds a different kind of day meaningful, although many of us do things that a lot of people like to put in their day.

Imagine if you wanted a meaningful day, as we all do, but you had no way to make that happen for you. If you have no speech, or if your speech is echolalic, repetitive, or very difficult for others to understand, it would be extra hard for you to engage others in putting together a meaningful day for you. And don't be fooled into thinking we don't all need cooperative people to put together our meaningful day. Just consider how many people you have contacted or will interact with to make today a day with meaning. Just your reading this text has required a bevy of circle members, editors, designer, printers, publishers, distributors, a library system, bookstore or online store, and the people who recommended it to you. And that is just one thing you will do today with meaning for you. Real independence is an illusion, a media hype of Marlboro men. We are all totally interdependent on everyone else around us.

If you were physically unable to move or to express yourself in typical ways that convey meaning to others, that would put a lot of barriers between you and what you want in your day. If your cognition or perceptions are different and you haven't the ability to let others know and understand that, that too can put a big crimp in your having a meaningful day. If you live with tremendous anxiety that conflicts with your delight in the everyday, that certainly can get in the way of having a meaningful day.

Often people living with these and similar impediments have had little opportunity for meaningful activity in their days. Like Mike, who wrote a short and telling book about his early years, they might spend their entire childhood and adolescence in a bed counting cracks on an institution's ceiling. Or after they got out of school, if they were lucky enough to have been in school, they could spend the bulk of their day sitting by a window, or in front of the tube. It is OK to watch TV if it is a chosen part of your meaningful day, but to sit incessantly in front of soaps or game shows or CNN all day could make anyone deathly bored or edging toward violence.

There is a strong push in the personal futures planning movement to work toward developing meaningful days for people living with varying types of disabilities. Too many people have spent too many years in inactivity, bored literally to death, in institutions, or in the back rooms of their families' homes.

Let's go back to what your meaningful day looks like. How did you figure out what would make it meaningful? Trial and error? Probably. As you grew up, and went out, you tried many activities, and inactivities. Your family and friends exposed you, and you them, to many new experiences that you could try, to see if those activities brought pleasure, productivity, peace, purpose, creativity, energy, etc. into your daily life. It made for a broad palette of experience that you could draw from to put meaning into your day, and bring meaning into the days of those close to you.

Now imagine that the way you perceive novel things and experience them is somehow very frightening, producing for you a lot of anxiety around new experiences. Putting meaning into your day will be very difficult if it involves changing a carefully constructed routine that assures that no threatening new things will suddenly intrude. And yet, like anyone, you still want pleasure, productivity, creativity, etc. in your life. How could you move beyond the terrible anxiety to bring more meaning into your day? How, with the limits you have to your expression in speech, and to your understanding of what motivates others around you, could you help others to know what they could do to bring meaning into your life?

Well, it isn't easy, and Raymond had to find a lot of ways to teach his group what made his day meaningful and what didn't.

First case in point

When Betty first met Jo Ann and Hope and Milton, they began to look at Raymond's day and what they could do to make it a richer day for him. At that time Raymond's primary activity was watching TV. He filled the rest of his day with frustration, harassing his parents, doing errands with his mom when she could pry him off the sofa, and drinking Pepsi. Even moms can run out of ways to motivate their young people, especially when a dense atmosphere of tension and anxiety has built up around any possibility of change.

Betty said, "When we first got the group involved, Milton stayed up all night thinking up things for Raymond to do."

So Milton would put two and two together:

"Raymond loves TV; he loves handling and using his remote control. How can I make that a richer experience without going too far into Raymond's anxiety at new things? Of course! Nintendo!"

Milton rented a Nintendo game. These were the early days of video games, mind you. Milton brought the Nintendo game over and showed Raymond how it was played.

"See, Raymond? Here is the control, just like your remote, and you move this around to make it move on the TV. C'mon, you want to try it?"

"NO!!"

"Well, just watch me for a little bit."

"NO!!"

Something about the Nintendo was very uncomfortable for Raymond. He didn't have a way to tell Milton what bothered him about the game, but he knew how to let Milton know he didn't want to do it.

"It probably wasn't a good idea," Milton admits.

"It made him angry; it was using his TV. It required fine motor control and he couldn't do that. And he didn't like it. But I pushed it on these two issues and despite several tries I finally gave up attempting to put meaning into Raymond's day with Nintendo.

"He can't get out into the community if he won't get off the couch. He's got to get off the Haldol. It's like you've got to be able to converse and move. And I was so driven to do things and Raymond was so not in a place to do new things. I think Betty was really wondering about me.

"But he still let me come back three or four times after that, I think. He'd say, 'Do you still have the Nintendo, Milton?' And I would say 'no' and then he would let me in."

"Had you said yes he would have said, 'I'll see you later,'" Tim comments with a laugh.

Betty adds, "I think Milton was ingenious to come up with some of these ideas. One day he said, 'Well, Raymond, if you don't want to do what I want to do, could I do what you want to do?' Raymond would go to the grocery with me. So Milton took Raymond to the grocery, and that's really what broke the ice with Milton. And to think Milton stayed up all night to think of this."

"Working on 'his' common sense. Right!" laughs Milton at his own expense.

Second case in point: Trial and error

Because Raymond had spent most of his days on the couch with his TV, he was more hesitant about walking very much at this time. Going for a walk would be a rather threatening experience. There would be new things to see; new sidewalks to navigate. You might run into other people. Raymond didn't encourage this novel experience.

Raymond's group felt that he needed to have new experiences to build up his tolerance for them. They thought his hesitant walk was keeping him from getting out. Someone suggested Raymond look into getting a scooter. Team members sought out medical suppliers, and other stores that handled scooters. Raymond and his sister Carolyn actually went out to Biggs to try out a scooter in the store. He enjoyed it. The doctor sent a requested verification of need. Everyone was poised to get Raymond the scooter.

In three more months the scooter became a dead issue. Raymond was too busy trying other new things and was walking without difficulty and getting around a whole lot better.

Raymond's family and friends learned quickly from Raymond that they could do new things with him, gradually, and often in the context of old familiar experiences. They realized that you don't tell Raymond to do a lot of new things at once, especially when it isn't his idea to do it.

Third case in point: Trial and success

Raymond met his friend Nancy while not having lunch with her in a McDonalds with Milton. "Don't you want to meet Nancy?" Milton asked Raymond, after he had arranged for them to meet Nancy there.

"NO!!"

"So we just sort of waved at each other across the dining area."

But this was to be a fast and happy relationship. Nancy worked with Milton on developing employment opportunities for people. She found a volunteer position for Raymond at the Highland Presbyterian Church, which eventually became a paid job for him every Friday. Raymond liked the people at the church right away.

Ruth Chaffens prepared the bulletins each week. Raymond and Jim would come into the nice shaded stucco house next to the big church at about nine-thirty and turn through the windowed doors into a big room off the central hall. Deep maroon carpet muted the sounds and the grasscloth wallcover made it a warm, rich kind of place to work. Ruth would set two parts of the bulletins out on the big table, usually the worship sheet and the announcements. She knew not to put more than two out, because Raymond handled two sheets best. He would get settled at the northwest corner of the table and, after a brief Pepsi and cookie break provided by Ruth, proceed to fill and fold each bulletin until he was finished. He did enjoy waving at other staff members and inquiring about their dinners the night before and how their cars were. But Raymond might have loudly objected if a church worker dared to come in and sit while Raymond was working.

"Raymond would shout out at first," Ruth said. "I would jump a mile and then settle back down. I wasn't afraid; I knew he wouldn't hurt me. It just took a little getting used to. And once he felt at home here, he was everybody's friend. Raymond was like a big teddy bear. He had such a wonderful smile." A small framed portrait of Raymond sits on the mantel over her shoulder in her office.

Ruth told about one day when Raymond had a difficult outburst. "He only did this once in the ten years he worked here. He moved the big oak table across the room and then knocked off the computer on the desk on one side. He left shortly after that."

Betty was very concerned about this outburst, because she knew just how much Raymond's job at the church meant to him.

"Barry called me up and said, 'I would like to ask Raymond if he wants to go apologize. Now don't say anything to him, Betty, until I come over.' [Barry Whaley is director of Community Employment Inc., which facilitated Raymond's work situations as funds for these came available.]

"When he came he said to Raymond, 'I wonder if you want to go see Ruth.' And Raymond said, 'I'll get my shoes.' He shot off that couch and went to get his shoes. When they got there he said to Barry, 'Don't say anything, don't say any thing.' Then Raymond apologized to her. That was one friend he didn't want to lose.

"We always wondered if Raymond's outbursts were willful or not willful. It seemed willful at times, but most of the time it really wasn't. It was his only way to handle frustrations."

Ruth remembered, "One Christmas I gave him a set of holiday suspenders. I had asked Jim if he wore a belt. I hadn't noticed. Raymond wore those suspenders for every holiday season after that for as long as he worked here."

This was real success. This job was part of a meaningful day for Raymond. And he worked at this job for ten years.

Fourth case in point: Success and burnout, Raymond and Jim

One way that the group found for Raymond to make his behavior manageable and to make his days valuable and full was to find a day habilitation supporter for him. Milton and Chuck began to introduce Raymond to bigger days, with more activities and tasks. When he seemed comfortable enough to make a day out in the community a regular thing, Jim Schrecker came to Raymond's day through Seven Counties Community Habilitation Program.

Raymond and Jim Schrecker began to spend time together in early 1993. Their association started off with a bang, since one day early in their time together Jim's car caught on fire and Raymond had to sit with the EMS people while waiting for Jim.

"I know one of the first places we went when we started spending time together was the old Hardee's down there on Bardstown Road near Weber Avenue," Jim says on the tape he sent from his home in the Philippines.

"It's not there anymore. That was a fun place, a place that Raymond enjoyed. Be fore we'd gone in there too many times, they started calling us by name. And we had little ceramic coffee cups, and on one side they said Hardees, and on the other you could put your name on it in indelible ink. We kept the cups for a while and then we lost them.

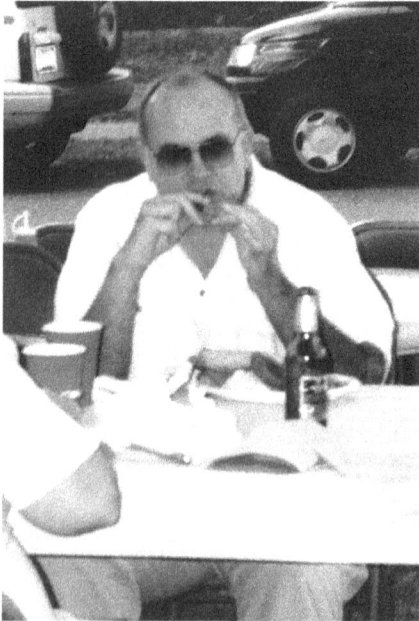

That made me feel like Raymond was at least open to new experiences and it encouraged me to go on and try to do some different things with Raymond that maybe he hadn't been used to doing before. And I was particularly happy that he would accept me taking him out and let me take him out in the community, not being a member of the family."

Raymond soon enjoyed trips to a gym with Jim, where he started out riding the exercise bike and built up to a weight-training routine. Jim and Raymond became Kentucky Harvest volunteers, picking up goods at local food stores and bakeries and taking them to the Food Bank. Raymond continued his job with the Presbyterian Church, folding bulletins, with Jim's support.

In September of 1993, soon after they started spending time together, Jim and Raymond headed down the road for a camping weekend at Otter Creek Park. It had been a long while since Raymond's childhood camping experiences at Deam's Lake. Those had ended with some distress, so Jim was taking a gamble.

Jim Schrecker at a fish fry.

"It was great," Jim recalled.

"I called the director. Normally they want you to rent out the cabins for a couple of nights but I explained the situation and he let me rent a cabin for only one day and night. We cooked outside and inside both, I think. We did hamburgers on the grill outside, and frozen french fries inside in the oven and just had Cokes and potato chips and things that you would have for a picnic. We went for hikes on the trails near the cabin. It was very pretty. If you haven't been to Otter Creek, you ought to go there. But anyway, it was very interesting and I enjoyed it and I think Raymond enjoyed it too. There were absolutely no problems. I think it was a very successful endeavor with things that were a little bit unfamiliar."

The overnight went well. The cabin did have TV, a major comfort factor for Raymond. The next morning they enjoyed breakfast at the lodge before making their return trip. This had been a real stretch for Raymond and a success for both men.

The group felt that this boded well for future outings for Raymond as he got used to being out and on his own with a new friend.

The family was always looking for a personal physician for Raymond. Often medical personnel would only see Raymond once or twice before breaking off the connection. Jim took Raymond to his own doctor appointments to show him that there was little to be anxious about. Then when Jim had to be in the hospital, Raymond visited him and helped him with drinks. These reciprocal visits were good for helping Raymond deal with his strong anxiety about medical issues. This time spent with Jim in medical visits was a great help for Raymond tolerating the tension better when his father was in the hospital a few months later.

Jim added about the day-to-day with Raymond, "Well, shopping was always fun for Raymond because I would try to make situations where he was successful. For instance if we were going to go get a loaf of regular sandwich bread, we would go to the Kroger and go back to the area where the bread would be, and I would ask him, 'Raymond, help me pick out a loaf of bread,' and he would say, 'They are right there.' He would pick out a loaf of bread and I would say, 'Thank you very much.'

"Any time that I thought the situation could be successful, I tried to repeat those successes at least a couple times a day. Everybody likes to do well. It makes you feel good about yourself and what you are doing."

By June 1994 Raymond and Jim were visiting a bakery for Kentucky Harvest three times a week. They were at the spa doing weights several days a week. They worked at the Presbyterian Church stuffing bulletins on Friday. They bowled regularly, building up Raymond's scores. They started going to the EnTech Center at the Library to learn about computers. Raymond was attending Project Neighbor dinner evenings once a month, and they enjoyed doing errands together and often having lunch out. All of this required a lot of planning on Jim's part, with suggestions from the team at regular meetings.

In early 1995 the new owner of the spa told Jim that he would have to purchase a membership to continue coming with Raymond. That was prohibitive financially and no discussion with the owner seemed to mitigate the situation. The guys lost their spa time. That was a big loss for Raymond who had really come to enjoy his time at the spa.

June of 1995 marked a milestone for Raymond. He began spending four hours in the evenings with Owen McWilliams. This eased the situation at home, and brought more variety into Raymond's day. In the long run it became the stepping stone for Raymond's move out into the community. During this time Raymond and Jim continued to be a good team in the daytime.

By very early 1996, Ray was spending much of his day with Owen, Jim, and occasionally Tony. They were all doing things with Raymond that nudged him to more independent action. It was a rich time in Raymond's life. By June Raymond was spending twelve hours of his day out on his own with Jim, Owen and others. Nancy summed this up in one of her informative letters to the group:

"Jim and Raymond continue to be out and about, combining just hanging out together with various scheduled things such as volunteer work, errands and social times with Clinton, etc. Owen and Raymond are working on shopping and preparing simple meals and other things that will help prepare Ray for living in an apartment."

This time out extended into Raymond spending some time overnight with the McWilliams family, Owen, Julie and later baby Grace.

Owen describes their time together: "Initially on our days together I picked up Raymond and we went back to my apartment and hung out together. We'd go pick up Julie from work around 9:30 p.m. and drop Raymond off on the way home. Later, Saturdays were added and we'd hang out, make meals and eat, run errands and such. Raymond also spent a week with us when he wasn't getting on well at home."

Jim and Raymond continued working together for another year. Their time was doubled from four to eight hours daily. The long hours together probably took their toll and signs began cropping up that all was not going well in the relationship. Raymond and Jim began spending a lot of time at Jim's house, according to Raymond. Betty heard from Raymond that he was feeling nervous with Jim. She began to believe that planning for forty hours a week of day program was more than Jim needed to be doing. Raymond began expressing his frustration by pounding on the walls and dumping his TV sets at night. Betty considered asking Jim if he wanted fewer hours. She was thinking that he was not feeling involved with Raymond anymore. It was hard for anyone to think of closing out this part of Raymond's life and moving on.

Jim remembered, "Well, I don't know if he was getting bored with me, but things were changing toward the end of the four years. I tried to change some of our activities. We started going out to Gerald's house and visiting with him for a while. He was getting in a satellite TV or something and we would be talking about that, and he would show us what he was doing with that, and show us how he was working on cars and things. So I thought that would get us going in the right direction again, but still it seemed like he was getting bored with me or I wasn't coming up with enough different activities to keep him interested."

Jim had a lot of success with Raymond. But working one-on-one with a person who needs a lot of support to make his day worthwhile can take a toll. Perhaps it was hard for Jim to see that his forty-hour week with Raymond was burning him out. It was burning Raymond out as well. They were unable to find enough interesting activities to effectively fill forty hours. The strain was telling on both men.

"The great support that I had from Mom and Dad Atherton and Gerald and his sisters helped a lot," Jim remembers fondly.

"I always knew that they were there. All of them were always ready to give their opinions on what was happening and why and what else could happen. Without the family support there our work together wouldn't have lasted four years, or been nearly as successful as it was. I think Jim Atherton was getting ill toward the end of our time together. I don't know for sure if that would have affected Raymond being apprehensive. Maybe he was worried about that and couldn't express his feelings."

"One day during this time Raymond climbed slowly up the stairs to art therapy in an agitated state," Julie remembers.

"Betty accompanied him. He looked dark in the face and his eyes would roam up and seem to be stuck. He was shaky in his gait.

"While he had a bathroom break Betty talked about Raymond's state of mind and how distressed he was after having torn the mirror off of Jim's car. Raymond was angry with Jim and expressing it in ways he knew how. Betty was very concerned with the ambivalence of Raymond's feelings. Raymond sensed the tension building between himself and Jim. But at the same time he didn't want to lose what had been such a good and productive relationship in his life. It was this kind of double dilemma that made it particularly hard for Raymond to cope. At this same time Raymond's dad, Jim, was having serious health problems. Anxious about his father, Raymond would want to hang around home at the same time that his dad needed quiet and peaceful time. This layered another level of tension on Raymond.

"Betty was in the middle, needing to keep the home front peaceful for her husband, and having to keep Raymond at home on days he and Jim Schrecker weren't able to cope. Betty would stop Raymond from beating on the walls and doors. She'd say to Raymond, 'You'll be with me today, so you've got to cut the comedy.' Raymond would reply, 'I'll be good.'

"Nancy arrived for Raymond's art session shortly after Raymond had inhaled his Pepsi. He chatted a bit with us, but it was obvious he was agitated. Nancy noted that he was doing everything in double time. Her arrival seemed to calm him a little and he asked Betty if she would leave. She took a chair and sat outside the studio in the hallway. After she left, Raymond twice brought up that his mother was upset and that was worrying him. He knew things weren't going well. He went on and started his word and picture recognition pages. The routine of these projects settled him a little.

"Raymond took a bathroom break after his first pages and finding Betty in the hall, he asked why she was still there. She explained that she needed to stay in case he needed a ride. He was OK with that and continued with his break time.

"When Raymond returned we worked with sentences on sheets on the wall. He was able to match pictures with written phrases right away and was very pleased with himself. We 'high-fived,' and jumped up and down together to celebrate the success. He 'got a kick out of that,' he said and completed his task with pleasure.

"We sat down at the long table to make a decorative card to give to his Mom. We picked out pictures to add to the card. Raymond was now getting very foggy and more tired looking, having had two Haldol to begin with. He decided not to work on a second card for his Dad, and asked to use the computer to dictate one of his poems. When we turned it on he yelled out, 'Butt out!!' twice. Then to himself he yelled, 'Would you shut up!' He looked drawn and simply mortified. I asked him if he would like to go and get some rest. He was very relieved, having struggled to hold himself together to try to finish our art time. He said he was sorry he yelled.

"'Could we get together again?' Raymond asked.

"I said, 'Of course.' Raymond made a bee-line out the door and Betty drove him home.

"Nancy and I tried together to understand how Raymond's deteriorating situation with Jim could leave such a deep hurt. We could see the difficulty for Raymond in communicating that to people around him. We were both impressed that he held it together for this meeting and let us know that things were peaking before he couldn't control it any longer."

As Gerald remembers that time, "Raymond would let you know when he was not happy with things. You just had to be aware. I think the world and all of Jim. But Jim's life at that time was not conducive to flexibility. Things were changing for him.

"If I could say any one thing to caregivers, I'd say, 'You really have to be aware of the person you care for in their actions. If this person is throwing a fit, regularly, why?'

"No one seemed to understand why Raymond was going through this phase. Finally one day I came over and said, 'Mom, there is something going on with Jim that Raymond doesn't want to be with him right now.' Mom then told me how Jim's life was changing; that they were spending most of their time at Jim's. And Raymond wasn't happy doing that.

"I hurt Jim's feelings." Gerald said sadly. "I said, 'Jim, just leave. He doesn't want to be around you.'

"Jim obviously cared deeply about Raymond. I know it hurt for him to hear that. It shouldn't have escalated to that level. Things had changed in Jim's life. We could have learned from Raymond to be aware of his change in attitude."

Jim had a similar inability to tell what was going on with him and Raymond. Betty decided to take the transition into her own hands and contacted Rocky Robinson, Raymond's current case manager from Seven Counties Services. Raymond consequently had a "vacation at home," while people in his support group looked at and discussed changes to be made in his daily routine. By the next group meeting members were still finding ways to make this happen. The group formally thanked Jim for his good work with Raymond and hoped that he would remain in contact with Raymond, and with the group if he so chose.

Fifth case in point: More trials and more successes

After successes in jobs, like his church job, and his volunteer job for Dare to Care, Raymond and his group looked to stretch Raymond's skills with other work outside the home.

Another job Raymond particularly enjoyed was at Frulatti's, a small cafe in the

Mall. Pat Noland, who was later spending Raymond's day with him, found him this position. Frulatti's is a small counter-front, salads-and-sandwiches stand in a large food court at the Mall St. Matthew's. It was probably a real challenge for Raymond to get used to going to the large, noisy food court three mornings a week for his job. He and Pat would go through the two narrow metal doors behind the little counter to get to the work area. It was a small but quieter space to work in. Only the two little oblong port windows opened to the bustle and echoing voices in the court. There Raymond enjoyed the restaurant prep work. He liked putting big chocolate chip cookies on the sheets in preparation for baking. He was careful about removing grapes from the stems for salads. If Pat hadn't become ill Raymond might have stayed and enjoyed that job for quite a while. It was becoming obvious to the group that Raymond really liked some kinds of work.

After Raymond moved into his own home, the group began to look into new possibilities for work for Raymond. Everyone's favorite was the idea that Raymond and his brother Gerald set up and maintain a Pepsi vending business. It had all the elements that they would enjoy. Raymond and Gerald would go periodically and fill the machines and maintain them. Raymond would get to be around his favorite Pepsis, and bug around in the truck with Gerald, and Gerald with his mechanical abilities could keep the machines in top working order, and make contacts with other mechanics at their businesses to put one of Raymond's vending machines at their location. It looked like a winner. Milton was looking into the possibility of grant funding, which would be used as start-up financing for Raymond to purchase his initial machines and product.

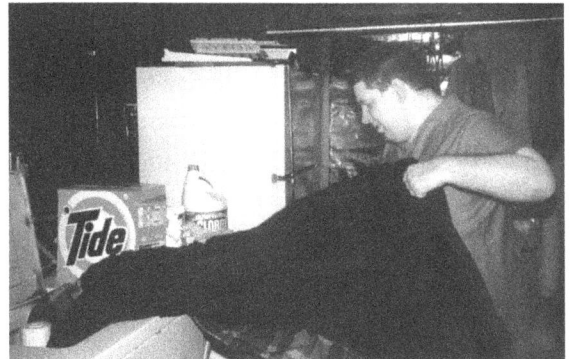

Raymond doiing laundry in the basement at his new home.

Having a productive and enjoyable day is everyone's desire. That isn't any different because a person lives with a disability.

"Something was said to me recently," says Milton, "that there is a big push and new dollars available to provide employment for people in day programs. And that is a really good thing. But people need to be clear about their motivation. Justice needs to be at the root. There's got to be more to their thinking than new funding for the service du jour. As services once considered radical, like supported employment, become more mainstream, the real challenge is finding and feeding the passion for the work to be done – just doing the right thing because it's the right thing to do."

Hope adds, "In Raymond's instance, there weren't other alternatives, such as work programs, day programs, that were OK. And certainly institutions as they were currently set up weren't OK for Raymond. If you work for justice, you work to figure this out. But you don't make any promises. But what drove us was the sense of the issue of justice around Raymond. Not just a belief in a model or person-centered planning technique."

Connecting with agencies

Even though Raymond's group was actually coordinating the services that they obtained for Raymond, it was necessary to work with agencies that offered some services, and primarily necessary to work with the Comprehensive Care Center that served as the pass-through for Raymond's Supports for Community Living funding. That agency was Seven Counties Services, the regional center for supports for Mental Health and Mental Retardation. Consequently it was necessary for Raymond to have a case manager from Seven Counties who worked closely with the group to help them use Raymond's funds to their best effect, and to avoid duplication of services with his other funding sources.

There was a long list of case managers/coordinators over the years because one of the problems with case coordinators is always turnover. People move through the system as staff even more rapidly than they move through as clients. It is hard for individuals to get used to the constant change in direction caused by fairly regular change in staff management. A consistent circle of friends buffers this fluctuation and makes for a more stable situation for a person. Without some consistency, and by only relying on a system, a person can become lost. Raymond had been particularly blessed with good case coordinators on the whole, some of whom stayed on as circle friends after they changed their work positions. Tim Estes and Linda McAuliffe are two examples.

Lee Bobzien was Raymond's second case manager after he had moved into his own home. She came on after Gwen Harbuck as case manager helped support Raymond and the family through his big transition. Lee, like Gwen before her, was particularly good at seeing how to balance the agencies, the group, and Raymond to make things work well for everyone. She also saw the differences that not having group support made for other clients she served.

Lee said, "My initial reaction to the circle and Raymond's situation was surprise at the level of support in his group, and the different directions and skills of all kinds of people who were offering support to him and to the family. You don't see that very often. You might see, instead, only an elderly parent or maybe a sibling stepping in if there is a problem.

"Fifty percent of the people I work with are in residential placements. There really is little in the way of futures planning going on for most of these people. And you really can't be ISP (Individual Support Plan)* coordinator and also do futures planning and do it right. In Raymond's situation his team was doing the futures planning, and doing it right."

Lee had the skills, as had Linda, Tim, Gwen, and others, to bring what was good from her agency and to make it serve the goals of Raymond and his group.

"It isn't the task of the ISP coordinator (case manager) to pull together a circle of support. It has to come out of the experience of the person, the family, people who get involved with the person, and other interested people who come together for this. The circle can be continually built by pulling in people who offer something to the team.

"The ISP coordinator can work with the circle, but isn't likely to be the one to bring it all together. As a family member your vision for your relative can be unclear. It helps to have a circle of people with more objective views to pull out possibilities for that person. It helps to have a care planner who can facilitate that bigger picture, elicit support from the group, and develop a program for the person out of that larger perspective."

And that is what Lee did, with a particular tenacity that made her a good part of this particularly tenacious team.

She continued, "It is important that the circle make a commitment to the person. What was different in Raymond's case was the level of committed involvement from the family. That made it easier for the circle to maintain their connection and their energy. When I was participating, I saw that Carolyn Wheeler was doing a great job of motivating everyone, as facilitator. But it was Betty's generous hospitality and of course Raymond's too, and that great pizza, that pulled us all together as a group. There was a social motivation there. People enjoyed each other's company."

Lee remembered, "Of course by the time I was on board, there were many results of a lot of hard work to witness. It was easy to see the benefits by that time. But I am afraid that Raymond's group was not the norm for a circle of friends. It was a real different entity. Perhaps seeing that this can happen around someone could encourage others to make it work for their people."

Which is what Raymond's circle would like to see happen.

"Raymond had a lot of people around him who had been 'in the system,' who weren't necessarily serving in that capacity for him, but who knew their way around the system, and how it could be made to work for him. It still wasn't easy, but it sure helped that they had a lot of know-how. People without that experience might be totally frustrated and say, 'Why can't this happen, and why not now?'

"Instead of fighting the system, Raymond's friends could work with it to get the best for him, and for everyone within the situation. That takes work, and time. A circle can make that happen for people."

Lee went on to shed light on the system's workings – and its problems.

"In the system, there is frustration because everything falls into categories with rules and regulations around them. For example, the SCL Waiver is not geared to serve people with a dual (concurrent) diagnosis. In fact there really haven't been residential services available locally for such people until recently a program opened in Shelbyville. We try to fit supports around people with dual diagnosis, but it is difficult. [Dual diagnosis, also called concurrent diagnosis, indicates that a person lives with a cognitive disability as well as a diagnosed emotional/psychological disorder.]

"For that matter it is next to impossible to get a diagnosis for a person in order to serve them properly."

Because the Medicaid system is medical model, nothing can be done for anyone without a medical diagnosis and prognosis to drive the services. Each person must be medically/psychiatrically evaluated and given diagnoses along the four Axes of the DSM-IV, or Diagnostic Statistical Manual, Fourth Edition.*

"Most diagnostic specialists don't take payment by Medicaid, and often avoid serving people with severe behavior issues."

But Lee reinforced the group's emphasis. "Besides, we know that it isn't the diagnosis that forms a person's life. It is the people around them. Currently the majority of dual-diagnosis people we serve are coming right out of an institution. Families often don't understand their deinstitutionalized relatives, and have no clue how to help them. Often a difficult and tragic situation caused them to separate from their relative in the first place. So you know they are going to be hesitant to get reinvolved in that person's life as supports. And they may be just making it day-to-day themselves. It is case by case, seeing if there can be family supports set up.

"Often by the time we see people, they are burnt out, as a family, in caring for their relative. They apply for the SCL Waiver to support needed services, but that is not a surefire fix. It is just a beginning.

"We go out to try to find appropriate providers to get services for the individual, and often we can't make things work with the provider effectively enough so that they can understand what they need to do to serve this person. There is training to do, and work specifically to see that the service is individualized. There is no cookie cutter to this.

"What was great about Raymond's family is that they stepped to the plate when it was time to work with providers. In Betty's case, family members were there at all times to offer support and intelligent back-up. Betty could address her family in ways that opened things up for Raymond, and when family members needed to move aside, they were able to without hard feelings or entanglements. Betty always listened to professionals, but then she took hold and made the appropriate moves."

Lee described how Betty's family moved in rhythm with hired staff to make things work for Raymond:

"Agencies that I work with are all willing to offer services to clients. The hard part is for the agency to hire appropriate staff to do the direct, hands-on work. You have to recruit the right people to work effectively with harder-to-serve people. It can be done. Raymond had good people working with him. Another part of the Raymond picture though, was back-up. The family was always there if need be. Staff knew that they could call on Gerald or Betty or others. They never felt that they were out there on their own. Perhaps that was the secret in Betty's family. She saw to it that no one was ever out there on their own with Raymond, perhaps because she had been and knew how difficult that could be.

"In order to work best with someone, staff need to know the person's history. They need to really know where the person is coming from. It helps to have as much of the big picture as possible in order to put things together effectively for the individual.

"Another thing that people may not realize is that things happen very slowly. Little things that happen can have great significance and should not be overlooked. Everything good that occurs takes place with baby steps. That was another of Raymond's family's successes. They were aware of the baby steps. They rejoiced in the little pieces as they would fit into the puzzle. Things never went unnoticed.

"Raymond's family embraced him and ran with his situation. They saw him as simply Raymond first. The challenges he offered were just part of who Raymond was. His family grew with the punches. They weren't into pity or martyr stuff. They were adventurous, always willing to try new things. In all of the time that I was working closely with them I never heard a negative comment about any ideas that anyone brought to the table. They honored all suggestions offered. Betty listened to everything, and then she would carefully weigh the ideas and use what might be of benefit.

"There was also a sense with Betty that you were the 'professional' coming in, but that you were welcome as a friend as well. The appropriate boundary was always honored, but the hospitality and warmth was ever present. No one was different and everyone was welcomed as they really were.

"Betty's family never gave up, no matter how hard things got. I remember going to HUD with Betty and Raymond when they were making applications for Raymond's house. Betty would do things like that over and over, no matter how frustrating it got to be. She knew that what she could do would make a difference for Raymond.

"Raymond enjoyed making things fun, especially one-on-one. I really liked when he came to visit me, and bring me art work that he had done, or those fabulous Christmas cookies. I'd always have a little snack for him. He liked that. But when things would go flying, and that seemed to happen in large groups for him, I worried about what was going on inside of him. At his home, he was so happy to show me around, and liked showing off his key chains. He was a good host and a fun guy.

"Maybe Raymond taught the family that depth of acceptance and hospitality to all. Or maybe it was part of the family already, and Raymond was lucky to be born into that gift of hospitality."

Raymond and his family were also particularly blessed with a number of case managers who were unusually gifted at what they did. While there was continual turnover of coordinators, most of them brought skill, sensitivity, and a lot of imagination to their work with Raymond. Another case manager who was one of Raymond's favorites, and served in several capacities while a member of the group, was Linda McAuliffe.

"I first met Ray and his family when Tim Estes, who at the time was facilitating the group, brought me into the group as a case manager. His job was changing at Seven Counties so I would be taking over the case management function. I realized quickly that my job was going to be a lot easier due to the range of activities and action steps performed by Ray's team. At the time I had over a hundred individuals with their names attached to my caseload so the group was able to accomplish things much faster than I alone could have done. I remember looking around the room and thinking that this collection of people really was the Who's Who in the field of developmental disabilities in Kentucky. I felt honored to be a part of such a strong, cohesive, and committed group."

Since Linda spent time with Raymond as case manager, facilitator, support for day activities, and eventually Supports for Community Living administrator, she had a lot of views of Raymond and his situation.

"What made this group tick?" Linda asks and then answers: "The person at the center, Raymond. As I started to get to know Raymond, I saw a young man facing many inner struggles with feeling, thought, and emotions he often had no way to express. I watched him find ways through questions he had in his repertoire, through smiles and laughter, through jokes, and sometimes by shouting out his point. Often when he couldn't find the words he really meant, he used other words he knew that had elicited responses before."

Later Linda got even more involved in working on Raymond's team.

"I took a more active role in Raymond's life using my skills, and became facilitator for his team. I was recommended for that by long-time team member Nancy Brucchieri. I also spent more time with Raymond when I accompanied him to his appointments with art therapist Julie Cole. Through this experience with him I started to see how much we had in common. We hate crowds; we watched our fathers suffer through illness and death; we are hurt and confused when people don't do what they say they are going to do, and we struggle to find ways to express our deepest emotions. I was working on my MBA at the time and Ray never failed to ask me how my classes were going or if I had finished the homework I'd been putting off! As my work changed, my role evolved into a friend and team member. As part of the Supports for Community Living staff, I could offer assistance and support when it came to making this funding source fit into Raymond's life. I also assisted throughout the years in helping to figure out Supported Living. I've been known to write a letter or two in my time with Raymond!"

Linda felt the same connection with Raymond's group and with his family as so many others in the circle felt. "I felt as welcomed by them as I do with my own family. They have celebrated my successes with me as much as I have celebrated Raymond's with them. In fact, when I finally received the copy of my MBA degree, they were the first people to see it and share my triumph with me. In being a part of Raymond's life and his team, I have received much more than I could ever give."

So it took a combination of Raymond's family, his group, staff members recruited and hired by the group, and the support of case coordinators assigned through his Supports For Community Living to make his day, each day, meaningful to Raymond. There were years of tinkering and experimenting and trial and error efforts, but the outcome was days well spent, and interesting prospects for future work.

Chapter 14

The System?

Some thoughts on what the system offers

The people crowd into the small classroom and sit around the rather inaccessible U shape of shoved-together tables. Walking people and chair users mill around, filling the available space. Everyone watches as the energetic lady in the front of the room beams at them, engaging their interest.

"I am sure most of you have experienced the kind of professional disengagement that I am going to describe, but I hope to show you workable examples of service provision that I have personally seen benefit people who have what is often called 'dual diagnosis,' and now called 'concurrent diagnosis,' meaning mentally retarded with emotional and behavioral problems."

Beth is the presenter, vibrant and lively and keeping the audience at her fingertips even when the subject matter is essentially frustrating.

"Serving the difficult-to-serve, people living with the stigma of 'behavioral irregularities,' is a challenge for any service providers, and frankly most opt out. They don't want to deal with people who exhaust their already worn-out staff. Because of some clients' erratic behaviors, the issues around liability to staff, to consumers, are more than most agencies want to deal with. Consumers and their families and supporters struggle with a constant fear of disengagement from services. Families feel that agencies are disloyal and they become discouraged.

"There is little help or support from the medical community. Families seeking emergency help from local hospitals are often hustled off to the state psychiatric facility with great speed, even though that is not what they want for their family member.

"This becomes a community problem because the services are so intermingled in a person's life. If a day program refuses to serve a person, that can leave the person's residential program in jeopardy. Residential programs as a rule don't care for people during the day. If there are no residential services available then that person may end up in a state facility anyway.

"Many agency people are in over their heads. They simply don't know what to do. They will tell families, 'Your person doesn't fit. We don't know what to do for her. We can't support her.'

"Or providers will be proactive and set up meetings to talk about reinventing the system, industry wide, to develop appropriate wrap-around supports for these people. And then there is the treatment disconnect. The people used to working with people with mental retardation are not in sync with the people who treat emotional and mental illness. They don't understand each other's approach. They don't understand how to develop a good diagnosis. And without a good diagnosis, how can you treat appropriately?"

Julie, the art therapist, was attending this workshop, and she had this to say about the conundrum of "service provision" to people with multiple disabilities:

"At this point in the presentation I came a bit unglued. I was interested in what Beth had to say, because I respect her work, and all that she does by training direct service people who work in the field and by supporting self advocates. But at this point I realized that what wasn't making sense for me was that the approach that she was discussing was, of course, based on the medical model of service delivery. You diagnose – then you serve. This is the model followed by Supports for Community Living providers, under Medicaid. And in most cases "serve" has meant involvement in an institutional or community program with set circumstances and routines in which a participant or client must fit to be served. Again it is a diagnose/treat model that medicalizes people's lives."

But as case manager Lee Bobzien said in the previous chapter, getting an appropriate diagnosis is a very difficult matter. It is almost impossible to find diagnostic specialists who take Medicaid, or who want to serve people with multiple disabilities. Without the diagnosis a person cannot be slotted into the current service provision system. What is required is often unobtainable.

"In Raymond's situation and that of numbers of other people with concurrent disabilities, a careful, complete diagnosis was never a reality. Betty had been seeking out medical help since Raymond was an infant. She had only found one doctor, Dr. Roth, the neurologist, who had offered her consistent support," Julie noted.

"Pervasive Developmental Disorder" was the diagnosis Herb Lovett suggested for Raymond after he had met him. What does that mean, and how would that improve one's treatment?

Raymond was evaluated by Seven Counties and received the needed diagnosis. Lee Bobzien, one of his case workers, also said that one's diagnosis could affect the level of services (and the funds) you receive from Medicaid. The Supports for Community Living service levels are numbered from one to five and are based on physical, emotional, cognitive and behavioral impairments. Raymond had a high level of need on that basis because of his apparent cognitive level, his behavioral problems, and his need for some help with activities of daily living. In that way his "diagnosis" would affect availability of supports to him. He might be bumped higher on a waiting list for a particular service, if he were to seek that kind of assistance. This is an issue that needs to be looked at when a circle of support approaches the system for services for their friend.

How do you find out what services are available to a person in a community? How does one go about accessing those services? And if those services are paid for by Medicaid, how do you get an appropriate diagnosis, which is a prerequisite to that funding? For that matter, do you want to go to what is out in your community or rule those services out and develop your own supports? It is easy to get lost in what feels like a hopeless maze.

Despite initial frustration for Betty when she approached Seven Counties for services, with the group as supporters, she was able to get an appropriate evaluation for Raymond. Seven Counties assigned case workers who would work with the group to make things happen for him. This was necessary since Seven Counties is the funding agency for the Supports For Community Living funds (Medicaid).

There is a "system" out there, but it isn't some great bureaucracy so much as it is people trying to make difficult-to-provide services available in what can be very convoluted processes. If you approach this as solving individual problems with solutions from individuals, it seems less daunting and hopeless. It is better to network and talk to others in similar situations, or who have served others in such circumstances. It is better to seek peers who have gone through these experiences and ask them to show you the ropes, or to get in the boat with you and show you how to row.

Work?

Employment Services

As an example, let's look at what are called employment services, day services, or day programs. When a person with disabilities finishes school (and under IDEA* all people with disabilities are eligible to public education in the least restrictive environment possible up to age 21), what opportunities are available to that person to build a living?

If they were fortunate in their school situation (which many people like Raymond, living with concurrent diagnoses, are less likely to be), they might have been involved in a transition program which gave them training in a job setting of their preference.

Milton Tyree tells stories of staff on transition teams not seeing the forest for the trees, missing what might be the central interest and skill of a student because of a set of assumptions about his or her disability. The assumptions mask the young person's actual skill. A young man in love with computers who fiddles and troubleshoots in the labs of his high school is skipped over when it comes to placing him in a computer-related job. The transition coordinator saw his label of autism first, and didn't coordinate with teachers who appreciated the young man's skills as a *de facto* aide in their computer classes. It took an outside team to make the connection and to encourage the school to direct his transition process along the lines of computer technology.

Several friends with cognitive disabilities transitioned right from high school into jobs in hospitality/food service or the grocery field or the shipping industry. They are still with their original employers over fifteen years later. In fact one gentleman worked for a grocery company that closed. A new grocery company came in town to buy out the old chain, and he was hired back. That chain unfortunately also closed. A third grocery then hired him. His reputation as a steady, hard worker has followed him.

One of his friends has worked at her grocery since high school, over fifteen years. She walks to work each day. Another gentleman has held a steady job at a local restaurant for over seventeen years. He loves his work and has a long commute by bus morning and afternoon. Still another man has worked at a country club for over fifteen years and rides his bicycle to his job. In the past these valued workers may have been institutionalized, or be simply hanging around some relative's home, essentially ignored. But transition programs and family supports that took their skills and interests into consideration placed them in jobs in which they've succeeded.

Some people may not have the physical or cognitive capability to allow that more independent level of work, but they may do well in an organized work program which gives them meaningful work that satisfies them, challenges them, and pays a reasonable wage. One program in our area offers interesting and satisfying work for people who enjoy being outdoors and working with nature. They work on a horticultural team that develops and maintains landscaping for area businesses and individual customers. That type of program is different from the old workshop model which pushed production in a quota-driven situation, and which many participants found boring and stressful.

Others may enjoy a day program which provides a variety of activities of a work, recreational, and educational nature plus opportunities for volunteering. This type of program is rather rare, and waiting lists are long. Other day programs with long waiting lists include community-based days. These are usually centered in one location and participants go out into the community with program staff to do volunteer work, visit organizations, participate in community activities, and just do fun and interesting things on occasion.

Those are some options available in the system for people living with disabilities to enjoy work satisfaction, or an interesting, valuable day. Those options are often not available to someone like Raymond, who needed more support during his day, but would have liked to enjoy similar activities. For Raymond's group this was a challenge that they solved by adapting funding for day services to pay a community support person to make a valuable day along with Raymond. This included Raymond's part-time clerical job at the Presbyterian Church, and later his food-service job at Frulatti's.

One persistent frustration for the group was finding creative people to help build that valuable day, and to keep Raymond's time with his day support people interesting and fresh.

Residential services

Since the usual residential options available in the community literally opted out (by signing non-service disclaimers) of serving Raymond, the group had to skirt around the system and make a residential opportunity for Raymond on their own, while using appropriate funds to make this a reality for Raymond in his duplex apartment. This was the group's and family's preference anyway. Raymond eventually had all of the benefits that the system could offer, but only because his family and his support group had found access to the system in non-traditional ways.

Looking at a proposed service provision innovation

The current political climate is certainly not amenable to looking at independent living for people with disabilities. Or is it?

There actually is a push in some state governments, long touted, long awaited, to encourage a more independent way of life for people with disabilities. In Kentucky one program addressing this is called Consumer Directed Option* (CDO), part of the Kentucky Independence Plus Program.*

"The Kentucky Independence Plus Program is part of the National Cash & Counseling Demonstration Program* which allows Medicaid members who require waiver services to purchase those services differently. The program is a joint effort between the Department of Medicaid Services, the Department for Mental Retardation, and the Division of Aging Services." (http://arcofky.org/CDO/index.html)

If you are eligible to receive funds that can keep you out of institutional care and out in the community – such as Home and Community Based Services; Supports for Community Living; Acquired Brain Injury Services, or 1915c Medicaid waivers for those who are at risk of life in an institution – then you can opt for this CDO. This option will allow an individual to use Medicaid funds, to be allotted on the basis of a detailed plan of care showing how needs will be met for a year. The person can then hire staff and purchase services to meet independent-living goals.

For some people this is a dream come true. People have worked hard to make this option available. This will allow people who are ready for more independence and can make decisions for themselves the option of hiring whomever they want for their attendant care, homemaking, personal care, and respite care. Those are the covered services in this part of the waiver.

It will allow people who have concerned people around them willing to administer this program to hire people who will offer these services: respite, community living supports, community habilitation (day services, whether supported employment or day activity program, or a companion with whom to spend one's day).

This is essentially what Raymond's group did. They connected with agencies and individuals who could offer services that suited Raymond's needs. They supported the family in hiring and monitoring all people working with Raymond, and they worked with agency staff whose agencies acted as pass-through for the Medicaid money that funded these services for Raymond.

This worked for Raymond because he had truly dedicated family members who rallied around him and supported his every need. They were flexible and capable and deeply concerned that Raymond do well. They pulled support around themselves by offering hospitality and connection, and the network of friends that they had gathered worked well for them.

At a meeting Julie attended in which state representatives explained the CDO to consumers and family members, there were many questions that indicated a lot of concerns around the concept of self-direction for needed services. Julie reported:

> During the meeting I was sitting with Anne Scott, who is also a volunteer advocate overseeing her friend's situation for the long term. As we listened carefully to the trainers we agreed that this could be a good program, if somewhat complicated by the state supports involved, if there were families and volunteers ready, and competent, to provide such back-up.
>
> When it was question time during the workshop, the participants seemed to focus primarily on their own sense of lack of support. One mother was nearly in tears describing her son's needs and her sense of being overwhelmed by those needs and not having any support system to help her coordinate services for her child. As a new person in town she didn't feel she could pull together the team she would need to put all of this in place. She could see that it would be best to be able to choose what services he could receive, but she didn't see how she could work full-time, care for him all of the rest of her time, and also coordinate the services and monitor the funding and the direct service provision. It would be more than working three full-time jobs.
>
> Other family members at this workshop expressed similar fears and doubts. Anne and I both wished that the trainers could have been more clear that this program was new and only an option for Medicaid recipients. The way they presented the program emphasized this option as new and better, but also as less an option and more the direction that Medicaid would go in the future. The responses of the consumers present showed that some felt that this was good for a few and others felt it was too scary for most.
>
> We left the meeting frustrated that a program that could be ideal for many individuals and families, like Raymond's family, might simply be unusable by many because it seemed too complicated and difficult for most of the participants who were simply overwhelmed by the material at this training.

CDO offers contact with a support broker who is supposed to be available to a number of families 24/7. In the training, the implication was that this person would help you to develop your plan of care and from that develop your support spending plan. This broker would also show you how to complete all the forms necessary to file this information with Medicaid. This support broker then goes on to represent the individual with disabilities, although what that implies is not detailed. The broker is then to assist with the development, revision, and monitoring of an emergency back-up plan, in case the plan of care and support spending plan don't work out. The broker is to provide education and information to the person or family on self-determination and community resources, and to assist with recruiting, hiring and managing employees of the individual and negotiate pay rates with those persons. After all that is done, then the broker has the ongoing role of assisting with all paper-work and the CDO process, coordinating all the services for that individual served, and being accountable to the individual, the support people around that person, and the state.

The CDO is apparently setting up an agency which will provide these brokers to people living all over the state.

In Raymond's group, several people served as family brokers over the years. Nancy worked at it probably the longest. She was not working for the state at that time and played the role by ear, since there was no real precedent for it. She coordinated Raymond's support meetings, and often facilitated them during that time. She worked with other group members to support Betty in making grant applications for funds to hire and pay day habilitation people at first, and then respite and home habilitation support. Nancy was back-up in emergencies for the family and often took Raymond to art therapy and other appointments.

"I don't want to seem skeptical, but I think it will be difficult to hire someone from an agency to be all the things that Nancy was as family support broker," Julie said.

CDO will require that each individual participating have a volunteer representative. This will limit applicants to the program. The good thing is that the representative will be chosen by the participant and can be anyone that they choose. The bad thing is that so many people with disabilities live in isolation without a lot of family and social contact, and that lack will make it difficult for them to find a person to act in this capacity. It is a well known truism that many people with disabilities primarily have paid "friends," and few chosen ones.

This volunteer representative's responsibilities include recruiting, hiring, firing and supervising your staff, on a day-to-day basis. The state is assuming that people have friends or family with the capacity to do these complex tasks while effectively working with the assigned family broker.

Granted, this is an optional program, and it is ideal for those people whose circumstances make it possible, but it could only be beneficial to those few people. Maybe it is intended as a pilot so that young families with members living with a disability can see that there may be new ways to live more effectively.

Programs that don't seem to work

For people who live with serious cognitive or physical disabilities (or both) that preclude their being able to work in typical jobs, a day program is an alternative, but one that varies a lot in quality

Unfortunately, most day programs are primarily custodial in nature and often exist to serve elders but do so in a less than ideal manner. Here is a "virtual" tour of such a program that Julie visited while searching for appropriate day services for a friend:

> I arrived at the front door of a former retail establishment in a neighborhood strip mall. The large glass windows mean a bright and open appearance inside; it is in a neighborhood where many people may be going in and out give it a a lively ambience.

> Then again, this may be a failed retail area where there is no traffic or activity. Because of limited funds, a service program would seek out low-rent property.

> I was invited in by a worker and saw that the front area was arranged with round, covered tables. A television played in the background. Several people were sitting at the tables. Some were watching TV. Attention had been paid to making the room cheery with bright colors. But little seemed to be happening, and the TV droned on uninterrupted.

> The worker told me that this is the activity room (despite the lack thereof) where the participants meet, plan their day, eat meals, play games and generally hang out. Probably hanging out is the primary (non-) activity.

> She took me into the next room. It too was quite large and there was a U-shaped area of mismatched but comfy looking sofas in the center. A man was asleep on one of the several sofas, and the ever-present TV played in the top of the U. The worker told me that people like to relax here and watch TV and have down time. I was concerned that there might be a lot of down time.

> On one end of this room was a door to an area outside. We walked into a small courtyard, fenced and locked, containing three small picnic tables. The lady told me that participants enjoy spending time here on pretty days. But this whole time she hadn't told me anything about what spending time meant at this program, other than literally spending time.

> I decided quickly that this was not an appropriate program for the person for whom I was exploring programs.

> When you're checking out a day program for someone, go out and really take a look at it. Take members of your group. Don't accept less than what you want for the person you are supporting. Build your own "program" if what is available doesn't meet your standards for a good day for your friend or family member.

In Raymond's case, there was rarely any talk of "programs"

Raymond's circle assumed from the beginning that his day would be his own. His needs for supervision and companionship, because of his anxieties and unanticipated outbursts, warranted that Raymond spend his days with a friend. So Milton, Chuck, Tim, and Jim gradually got Raymond interested in being out and active for a day with them. Owen and his family helped make Raymond's evenings comfortable.

After moving into his apartment Raymond was spending afternoons with Sarah Tackett, shopping, cooking, and occasionally visiting his friends in the Dreams With Wings*residential program He particularly enjoyed the trip to a neighborhood fishpond where he could feed the fish and visit with other passers-by. Raymond and Sarah together built a shelf for his room where he could display his Pepsi and M&M collectibles. Raymond at this time spent mornings with Alex, his other day companion, doing things they enjoyed doing together: chores, shopping, visiting friends and family, and activities around town.

"This book is about possibilities." Julie says.

> I have had many mixed feelings as we wrote it, because while the possibilities played out in our friend Raymond's life, it was only "by the hardest," as my mother-in-law used to say. It was only by the strongest intention, the widest attention, and the deepest devotion that the things described in this book came about.

> Things like this worry me, because in my experience not many individuals and not many families have these strengths to sustain them in the long effort that keeps dependent people as safe and independent as they can be.

> When I was first approached in 1984 to serve as a New Neighbors Citizen Advocate, I had a naive notion that people out in the community were going to volunteer for this position pretty routinely as people with severe disabilities were leaving institutional care settings. The young lady that I was recruited for would not then have been a good candidate for independent living. At the time I met her she had recently been removed from an institution by a new program for increased community involvement called New Neighbors. That program was an early form (in 1984) of the Medicaid waiver for community-based supports, now called Supports for Community Living, in Kentucky.

> She was attending a segregated school for children with disabilities. She had autistic behaviors and seemed mentally retarded and like Raymond lived with a stunning explosive disorder which she enacted on herself and others with no apparent known stimulus. Unlike Raymond she had no known family or any community support.

> I was asked to become a guardian for this lady. A guardian essentially oversees the life circumstances of another person who has been judged to be unable to do

this for herself. The guardian makes decisions for another person about housing, employment, day program, or activities, and all financial, legal, and healthcare decisions that must be made.

So, having a guardian is not really independent living, although living in a home in the community is a part of independent living that is important to most people moving out of institutional care. Unless a guardian is motivated to see that a person's situations are as autonomous and self-decided as is possible, in light of physical or cognitive disabilities, that person probably will not be living very "independently."

So over the past twenty-two years my friend has lived in foster families, one family hosting her for fifteen years. The situation was not ideal, but it was more like a typical life than she could have had in the institution.

With the support of a futures planning team we recently moved our friend into a home with two other ladies under the auspices of a community that serves people with mental disabilities in residences and in a day program for some of the residents. It may not be ideal, but she lets us know enthusiastically, that she loves it and would prefer to be there right now in her new house with her friends.

So is this idea of people with disabilities living in the community like typical people feasible? Probably. Consider that fifty years ago the vast majority of people with severe disabilities lived in institutions like state hospitals, nursing facilities and private asylums. There was certainly nothing visibly independent about those lives.

Julie continues:

In the neighborhood where I grew up, there was a private institution, right at the end of our street. It was then called The Home for Incurables. I wondered a lot about what constituted an incurable, as I walked past the high windows. In my childhood, I don't recall meeting any of the residents, even though we lived less than a block apart.

A few streets away a young woman lived out in the community with her mother. She was severely physically disabled with cerebral palsy. I vaguely recall visiting her with my mother when I was very little. I believe our mothers had worked together in a hospital at some time. Her name was Emma Louise; it was etched on the bottom of a heavy clay ashtray she had made and given to my mother. She was living in the community, but in the care of her mother. At that time there would have been no other way for her to be cared for in a regular home, and I doubt she went out much since I don't recall a ramp. There was certainly no accessible transportation fifty years ago. She probably was what some people might call a "back-room person," stuck in an inaccessible home with a loving caregiver.

I live in the same neighborhood today. The "Home" is now called Highlands Nursing and Rehabilitation Center. That is certainly a different emphasis. I am unaware of Emma's fate. But I was amused a few weeks ago when I got in my car and discovered that the curb corners of my street were being removed by jack hammers in order to replace them all up and down the street with curb cuts. This had recently been done on several other corners in the old neighborhood, but it has taken twenty-five years to get it done, since activists in our town pointed out the need for such accommodations for people using chairs at least that long ago. People using wheelchairs and scooters move about in our neighborhood a lot. Not only do people living at Highlands Rehabilitation nearby use chairs, but people living in the subsidized Highland Court Apartments for elders and people with disabilities, and at the Day Spring community, which is apartments for people with disabilities. People living in their own homes and apartments use curb cuts to facilitate their getting around to meet, greet, shop, and go to schools and work. People with disabilities are living in the community, working in the neighborhood, and taking public transportation. This is different from fifty years ago.

Is there a place for institutions? Some months ago I visited a friend in Central State Hospital. Yes, Virginia, there are still state hospitals. The ICF/MR* (Intermediate Care Facility for the Mentally Retarded) there is a bleak place. My friend has tried two different modes of semi-independent lifestyle. She lived in an apartment in a small community of people with disabilities. And she lived in a home with another person with disabilities with round-the-clock staff. Her emotional instability at that time made it necessary for her to take time out and reassess her ability to live "independently."

Friends don't want her to be in a drab empty hospital room, old, marred, and worn, where her neighbors run willy-nilly into her space at any time and steal whatever they want. I was in her room with her when this happened.

Other neighbors at the facility scream persistently and are moved from room to room by aides. As I left after one visit, a woman sat by the elevator door screaming and signing that two people had hurt her, and she showed off bruises on her arms and neck. Aides leaned, seemingly indifferently, against the far wall, ignoring her rage. Those aides are probably numb with the grief of these people and do what needs doing which is all they can get done. I have met caring and interested aides in that hospital and watched them work well with residents, but the overall atmosphere is sadness, frustration, and perhaps perceived abuse.

The hospital is what is available to people with concurrent diagnoses who do not have people in the community to guard them, or whose guardians have done all they can and are up against a rock of despair about providing care for their person in their illness and disability.

A couple of years ago another state institution was under fire for incidences of alleged abuse. Three hundred people with developmental disabilities live there. The state wanted these people moved out of the facility and into other circumstances. Will families and individuals step forward to make this transition work-able? Will groups of friends and supporters gather around each of these residents and work up futures planning maps to make the new situations the best they can be? In the "best of all possible worlds," perhaps this will occur, but I have my doubts about how effectively this will happen in Kentucky, although I am aware that several families, agencies, and individuals, including some of Raymond's group, are working hard to develop placements for some of the people leaving the institution. The ideal would be for each of those residents to have a family and/or friends that are willing to support them with the level of attention and interaction that Raymond's family gave to him.

I drive down the street. One of the ever-ubiquitous magnet ribbons graces the car ahead of me. At the light I read it. Its background is a multicolored jigsaw puzzle. The slogan reads "Autism Awareness." Is this the earliest part, just becoming aware that there are many puzzles to be explored, puzzles of how to survive, how to cope, how to thrive, and how to make the puzzles work?

I often feel that the general population has little investment in such exploration. I was talking with a friend recently who let me know how limited was her awareness of people with disabilities and their lives. Over and over people have said to me, "Unless disability impacts your life personally, you will pay no attention to it." What surprises me about this is that you rarely see an extended family that does not have someone living with a physical, cognitive, or emotional disability. How much impact is needed before awareness occurs, and change begins?

Chapter 15

Safely Home

Meeting 1/15/02

The cozy living room is filled wall to wall with every chair in the house. Raymond wields his remote at the big-screen TV as guests come in, climb over and fill the chairs. Elbow to shoulder or leaning against the big-screen tube, people catch up on post-holiday news as they wait for everyone to arrive. A big group is expected, including Sarah Tackett, Linda McAuliffe, Carolyn Wheeler, Lee Bobzien, Carolyn Stansbury, Gerald Atherton, Betty, Raymond, Julie Cole, Nancy Brucchieri, and Carolyn's daughters, who are taking Girl Scout cookie orders.

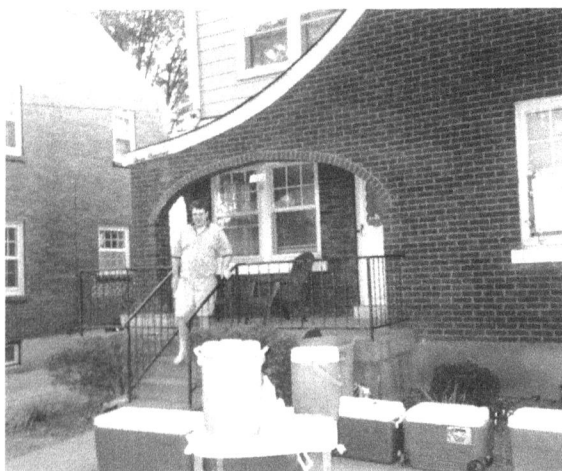

Raymond at home with fish fry preparations.

Two guests arrive. Becca Krall, Raymond's friend and former neighbor, is wearing her Supports for Community Living administrator hat. She has come, as has Vonda Vanderhorst, to look at how the Supports for Community Living and Supported Living programs mesh in Raymond's life. The delicate balance of the dollars that these two funding sources provide for Raymond's program must be carefully adjusted for him to have enough support in his home, and for his day to be successful.

The room is packed and Raymond is asking Betty if the pizza will be on time. She assures him that it will be. He asks several guests if they would like a diet Pepsi. Betty and one of her granddaughters hand in cold cans and napkins. The room is so full that people are passing the drinks around hand to hand. There is no lull in the several conversations going on at once.

Carolyn Wheeler calls the group to order, "so we can get some business done before we all end up with faces full of pizza." She welcomes the guests and everyone introduces themselves to refresh memories. Then Carolyn squeezes behind the recliner and readies her markers for the papers taped to the walls, as the reports begin.

Gerald tells the group, with his usual big grin, that Alex's friend Shawn is interested in getting to know Raymond better, to be a new roommate. Gerald is going to arrange some overnight visits to test "compatibility." Supported Living can pay part of a year's stipend for Shawn to live with and support Raymond at home. Gerald is working on dividing up the week's schedule to use the money effectively. The residential trainer position will be split between Gerald and the roommate. Becca tells the group that the grant was at 50 percent in December, so that makes it a half-year of funds left.

Because other people that have been hired to support Raymond had to drop out, Gerald feels that a new recruit needs to have a probation period before he gets a full stipend.

Vonda says to reapply April 1st for the next fiscal year. She says to apply at a higher funds level to meet the need for in-home support. Auditors reviewed all of the recipients of SCL and SL. Services cannot be duplicated, but SL can pay for approved non-SCL supports. Vonda doesn't see Ray getting service duplication, but that will be reviewed. The money he gets for residential support is not available through Supports for Community Living, which only backs staffed residences. SL encourages people to live in their own homes and funds that concept.

There are 1,900 people on a waiting list for this; people are trying to get services to as many people as possible. Carolyn W. says that there is a need to understand services person by person, not to exclude anyone from one program or another.

Milton and Barry will meet with the Small Business Development Center to develop a business plan for Ray's potential vending service. This is an exciting prospect for Raymond. He loves Pepsi, and traveling around. Raymond says he could "get a kick out of" a little vending business. Gerald, who is a mechanic, could place machines in repair businesses. He feels he could get several letters of intent from these businesses for machine placement. The machines cost $250 apiece. Betty's niece has two machines she would send for price of shipping. She realized $25 a week from her collections. Carolyn's daughter also made some spending money with vending machines.

There needs to be a police check on the potential roommate. Gerald said he'd find a company to do it on line, and he'll tell the new roommate, "You have to have insurance on your vehicle at all times and have a vehicle in good working order."

Ray had a good Christmas and delivered a lot of cookies. Betty said, "I credit this to Sarah. She planned a list with him and that took the tension out of it. He enjoyed the Christmas party at the Dreams With Wings house on Nanz Avenue. He played Santa." Raymond demonstrated his, "HO, HO, HO." It was impressive, room shaking.

The meeting ended with a sense of excitement. There were new things in the offing, a new roommate, perhaps a new job/business. It was a great start to a new year. Raymond smiled and joked as people made their farewells and went out into a crisp January afternoon.

Betty loved where Raymond had gone with her support and the support of his group. "The happiness in me is that Raymond worked and got the best. I loved how tall he stood and where he went. It is wonderful to think that his life just bloomed for him. Now Jim was more pragmatic than I was. He couldn't see that anything could work. But he is looking down and saw what happened. He was for anything we wanted and would back anything, but he sure didn't expect to see that happen."

This is a part of the story that we never thought would have to be told. At Ray's meeting on January 15 many of the gang were present and some guests. Ray was on his couch and king of his domain. It was a great upbeat meeting full of good news and new ventures. Ray was showing off his room decor which, with Christmas gifts in place, looked warm and homey and very Raymond. Gerald was excited about working with Raymond on his new vending machine business venture that Milton and Barry were looking into. The funds from Supported Living and Supports for Community Living were both in place and weren't conflicted in any way. Raymond had a new potential roommate who was beginning to visit and spend time with Raymond, and Gerald was planning an overnight for Ray and Shawn to get to know each other. Sarah and Raymond were having great times with their afternoons and their affiliation with the folks from Dreams with Wings. Alex and Raymond were having good mornings and meeting new people. Raymond's job at Highland Presbyterian was in great form. Betty said that he had his best Christmas ever. He had planned for it and really enjoyed it, especially when he played Santa for the Dreams With Wings party. Life was good, and it was continuing to get better.

For whatever reason the universe has, Raymond left us in his sleep, Sunday, January 20, 2002.

Rev. Tim Estes, in his warm and consoling eulogy said that Raymond's family and friends were never content with just what was for Raymond. They always hoped and worked for things to get better. They always succeeded.

Raymond Atherton: Reflections on his life
Tim Estes

I don't know how many of you recognized the song Carol just played, "Friends," by Michael W. Smith, but it is entirely appropriate for this occasion. The words are: "Friends are friends forever when the Lord's the Lord of them." You are here today as the forever friends of Raymond.

We're here to celebrate the life of Raymond Atherton. Even as we grieve his passing, we rejoice at the gift of having known him.

Raymond was, after all, a gracious host. Whenever we were at his house Raymond always made sure that everyone had a Pepsi. And for his friend, Tim, it was a diet Pepsi, because Raymond knew I shouldn't have sugar. He remembered, too, from one time to the next. That's a sign of a gracious host. But be forewarned because Betty has recommended to all of you that if you have stock in Pepsi you had better sell, because it is sure to go down now that Raymond isn't here to pass out Pepsis.

He also was quick to express his gratitude. Whenever you did anything for Raymond he let you know that he appreciated it. I remember when I took him to Sunday school at Beechwood Baptist, he said, "Tim, thank you Sunday school." We also went to eat at McDonald's several times, and he would say, "Tim, thank you McDonald's." Raymond always let you know that he appreciated what you did for him.

Then there were his disarming questions: "Where's your husband? Where's your wife?" and the ever-popular "Where's your car?" Our friend Milton Tyree pointed out that whenever he asked that question you always had to stop and think, "Hmmm, where *is* my car?" But when Raymond asked those questions it was his way of saying to you, "I care about you!" It was his way of showing his concern and friendship.

I'll quote my friend Milton again, because he was such a big part of Raymond's life. Milton was doing a workshop somewhere in Kentucky, and he pointed out to the group that one of the questions he always liked to ask while looking at how things were in the life of a person with a disability was the question, "How could this be better?" It's a great question! But someone in the group, a young lady, and I don't even know her name and wouldn't say it if I did, she asked an incredible question in response. She asked, "Yeah, but when does the better end?" In other words, when do we decide that everything is fine and we just quit trying to improve the lives of people with disabilities? Can you believe that question? Incredible, isn't it. But as I look around this room I see the people, his family, his friends, his advocates...I see the group of people who did more than any other group to make sure that for Raymond Atherton the better never came to an end.

I, for one, believe in a Lord who upholds that same purpose. That is why I believe today that for Raymond Atherton the "better" has not ended; in fact, for Raymond Atherton the "better" has just begun.

Raymond had a unique way of expressing his disapproval. I'm going to step away from the microphone because some of you know what is coming. But the first time I ever met Raymond was when I went to his support group. I said to him, "Raymond, I do a little work with Supported Employment, and what I would like to do is get to know you better, and look around in the community and find something that really interests you, and see if we can't get you a job."

Raymond let loose with a bone-shattering, soul-rattling, "NO!"

I said, "Uh...uh...well, okay..."

But today I want to say that I believe in a Lord who gives that same bone-rattling, teeth-chattering, soul-stirring answer in the face of death. "NO!"

God is the god of life. He is the God who has said "yes" to life in the person of the Lord Jesus Christ; a YES that resounds down the corridors of eternity, a YES that conquers the very reality of death itself. I believe in that Lord. I know Raymond's family does, too. And I know Raymond did as well.

And because I believe in that God, because I know that God is a God of life, I can say with assurance today that we who loved him will see him again. We can thank God for all of you who have been a part of Raymond's life, including the friends who are here today from Highland Presbyterian Church where Raymond worked in the office. And we can say with assurance that we will see him again.

I can say with conviction that Raymond is "Safely Home."

Safely Home

by Jon Mohr
(as recorded by Steve Green)

Children, precious children,
I know you're shaken,
a loved one taken,

Oh, but hear Me,
Come draw near Me,
Their pain is past now,
They rest at last now
Safely home.

They are strong and free,
They are safe with Me.

This life is merely shadow
Today there's sorrow,
But joy tomorrow,
Safely home

They are strong and free,
They are safe with Me.

One day you will join them
All together
This time forever.
Safely home.
Safely home

Afterword and Dedication

Raymond's life was shorter than anyone expected, but his group members have felt that he made a distinct contribution to the awareness of many people that people with complex concurrent disabilities can find a home in the community. He also taught us about the urgency of making this happen for people. We all learned lessons on seizing the day and living "thoroughly" from Raymond and his family.

Life is a cycle of growth and change and loss. During our time as a group together, and after Raymond left us, we experienced a number of losses of beloved group members and supporters. We wish to dedicate Raymond's book to Raymond, and to our colleagues and friends and loved ones who have gone before us.

Pat Noland

Toby Wheeler

Clinton Montgomery

Herb Lovett

Jim Atherton

Christine Kandler, "Meemaw"

Nancy Brucchieri

Tim Estes

Acknowledgments

Raymond's group would like to thank everyone who participated in the group's efforts to make life rich for Raymond. Most everyone was mentioned in the book, and we won't be redundant, but for all of you who were not, but know you were a part of Raymond's journey, we thank you from the depths of our hearts.

We'd like to thank Jack Pearpoint of Inclusion Press for encouraging our efforts, and for shedding light on the "whys" behind graphic facilitation as a vital tool in the futures planning process.

We also want to thank Mary Johnson and Barrett Shaw of the Advocado Press who carefully nudged us from early rough compilation to finished product. Their editing, formatting, and fine-tooth combing helped us pull Raymond's story together.

Appendices

Great ideas start new things happening. Most people who have great ideas have built those ideas out of experience, education, and awareness. We include these Appendices to provide some of each for people who will have new and great ideas for expanding and enriching the lives of everyone around them, especially people for whom great ideas were not thought feasible.

These appendices include resources and books from other people and groups whose ideas contributed to Raymond's larger life. Also included are primary sources on the groups' experiences with Raymond. The group decided to summarize tightly and include the minutes of Raymond's meetings over the years. We felt that had we such a resource when we started we wouldn't have had to invent so many trial wheels, which often rolled poorly.

We also include notes by Milton Tyree during his early experiences with Raymond. Again these notes can be mined for ideas on developing a new relationship in unusual circumstances. And there are summarized notes from Raymond's art therapy sessions, to illustrate Raymond's increased comfort with new things, and with communication skills.

Appendix A

Books suggested by members of Raymond's group

Bradley, Valerie, John Ashbaugh and Bruce Blaney, eds., *Creating Individualized Support for People with Developmental Disabilities.* Baltimore: Paul H. Brookes Publishing Co., 1994. P.O. 10624, Baltimore, Maryland 21285-0624.

Callahan, Michael and Bradley Garner, *Keys to the Workplace: Skills and Supports for People with Disabilities.* Baltimore: Paul H. Brookes Publishing Co., 1997.

DiLeo, Dale, *Raymond's Room: Ending the Segregation of People With Disabilities.* St. Augustine, FL: Training Resource Network Inc., 2007.

Etmanski, Alan, *Safe and Secure: Six steps to creating a personal future plan for people with disabilities.* Burnaby, B.C.: Planned Lifetime Advocacy Network, 1997.

Forest, Marsha, John O'Brien, and Jack Pearpoint, *PATH: A Workbook for Planning Positive Possible Futures.* Toronto: Inclusion Press, 1995. The Centre for Integrated Education and Community, 24 Thorne Crescent, Toronto, Ontario, Canada M6H 2S5, (416) 658-5363 or FAX 658-5067.

Girsch, Maria and Charles Girsch, *Fanning the Creative Spirit: Two toy inventors simplify creativity.* St. Paul, MN: Creativity Central, 1999.

Hildebrand , Adam J. , *One Person at a Time: Citizen Advocacy for People with Disabilities.* Baltimore: Brookline Books, 2004.

Holburn, Steve and Pete M. Vietze, *Person-Centered Planning: Research, practice and future directions.* Baltimore: Paul H. Brookes Publishing Co., 2002.

Kohler, Tom and Susan Earl, *Waddie Welcome & the Beloved Community.* Toronto: Inclusion Press, 2004.

Lovett, Herbert, *Learning to Listen: Positive Approaches and People with Difficult Behavior.* Baltimore: Paul H. Brookes Publishing Co., 1996.

Mount, Beth, *Dare to Dream: An Analysis of the Conditions Leading to Personal Change for People with Disabilities.* Manchester, Conn.: Communitas, 1991. P.O. Box 374, Manchester, CT 06040, (203) 645-6976.

Mount, Beth, *Life Building: Opening windows for change using personal futures planning.* Amenia, NY, 2000: Capacity Works.

Mount, Beth and Kay Zwernik, *It's Never Too Early, It's Never too Late!* St. Paul:The Minnesota Governor's Council on Developmental Disabilities, 1988. 370 Centennial Office Building, 658 Cedar Street, St. Paul, MN 55155, (651) 296-4018 voice, (877) 348-0505 toll free, (651) 297-7200 fax, (651) 296-9962 TDD, admin.dd@state.mn.us, www.mnddc.org or www.mncdd.org.

O'Brien, John and Beth Mount, *Make a Difference: A guidebook for person-centered direct support.* Toronto: Inclusion Press, 2005.

O'Brien, John and Connie Lyle O'Brien, *Implementing Person-Centered Planning: Voices of experience.* Toronto: Inclusion Press, 2002.

O'Brien, John & Connie Lyle O'Brien, *Members of Each Other: Building community in company with people with developmental disabilities.* Toronto, 1996: Inclusion Press.

O'Brien, John, Connie Lyle O'Brien and Gail Jacob, *Celebrating the Ordinary: The emergence of Options in Community Living as a thoughtful organization.* Toronto: Inclusion Press, 1998.

Pearpoint, Jack, *MAPS (Making Action Plans).* Toronto: Centre for Integrated Education and Community, 24 Thorne Crescent, Toronto, Ontario, Canada M6H 2S5(416) 658-5363 or FAX 658-5067.

Schwartz, David B., *Who Cares? Rediscovering community.* Boulder, CO: Westview Press, 1997.

Shaffer, Carolyn R. and Kristin Anundsen, *Creating Community Anywhere: Finding support and connection in a fragmented world.* New York, N.Y.: G.P. Putnam's Sons, 1993.

Smull, Michael W. and Susan Burke Harrison, *Supporting People with Severe Reputations in the Community.* Baltimore: Community Support & Access Unit, Department of Pediatrics, UMAB, 1991. 630 W. Fayette Street, Baltimore, Maryland 21201, (410) 328-2140.

Wolfensberger, Wolf, *A Brief Introduction to Social Role Valorization as a High Order Concept for Addressing the Plight of Societally Devalued People, and for Structuring Human Services,* Revised 3rd Edition. Syracuse, N.Y: Syracuse University Training Institute, 1998.

Appendix B

Glossary

ABC Theory

A theory or technique of therapeutic change developed by Albert Ellis in the context of Rational Emotive Behavior Therapy. Antecedent – Behavior/Belief – Consequence. This approach is used when assessing behavior and behavior disorders. What precedes the inappropriate behavior, what is the behavior and what will the consequence be for the inappropriate behavior. For example, a child begins rocking profusely in his wheelchair once the classmate that was helping him leaves. The antecedent is the fact that the child didn't want the classmate to leave him. The behavior was rocking in the chair. The consequence is something that needs to be put into the place to stop the inappropriate behavior. When special needs committees get together, they'll often refer to the ABC to help pinpoint behaviors to change. It's important to know what the antecedent is.

www.smartrecovery.org/resources/library
http://specialed.about.com/od/specialedacronyms/g/ABC.htm

A.D.A., Americans With Disabilities Act

The ADA prohibits discrimination and ensures equal opportunity for persons with disabilities in employment, state and local government services, public accommodations, commercial facilities, and transportation. It also mandates the establishment of TDD/telephone relay services

www.ada.gov/

Art Therapy

How Did Art Therapy Begin?

"Art therapy did not emerge as a distinct profession until the 1940s. In the early 20th century, psychiatrists became interested in the artwork created by their patients with mental illness. At around the same time, educators were discovering that children's art expressions reflected developmental, emotional, and cognitive growth. By mid-century, hospitals, clinics, and rehabilitation centers increasingly began to include art therapy programs along with traditional 'talk therapies,' underscoring the recognition that the creative process of art making enhanced recovery, health, and wellness. As a result, the profession of art therapy grew into an effective and important method of communication, assessment, and treatment with children and adults in a variety of settings. Currently, the field of art therapy has gained attention in health-care facilities throughout the United States and within psychiatry, psychology, counseling, education, and the arts. For more detailed information on the history of art therapy, please see AATA's publication list for A History of Art Therapy in the United States."

www.arttherapy.org/aafaq.html

Citizen Advocacy

C.A. is long-established program around the U.S. which matches capable interested volunteer advocates with individuals who need support in the community. Advocates may relate to a person as a guardian, a payee, a home provider, or simply a friend in an expressive relationship. An advocate looks out for the concerns of the individual with a disability as a family member would.

www.savannahcitizenadvocacy.org

www.councilonmr.org/ca.htm

C.D.O., Consumer Direction Option

"CDO is a new option that is being offered for Kentucky Medicaid Waiver members who are currently receiving or become eligible to receive Home and Community Based waiver (HCB) services through Kentucky's Medicaid Waiver program. CDO allows waiver members to choose who provides their non-medical waiver services which allows them greater freedom of choice, flexibility, and control over their supports and services. Members can choose to direct all or some of their non-medical waiver services."

http://chfs.ky.gov/dms/Consumer+Directed+Option.htm

The Community Choice Act of 2007

(S. 799 /HR 1621): A Summary

"The Community Choice Act gives people real choice in long term care options by reforming Title XIX of the Social Security Act (Medicaid) by ending the institutional bias. The Community Choice Act allows individuals eligible for Nursing Facility Services or Intermediate Care Facility Services for the Mentally Retarded (ICF-MR) the opportunity to choose instead a new alternative, "Community-based Attendant Services and Supports." The money follows the individual!

"In addition, by providing an enhanced match and grants for the transition to Real Choice before October 2011 when the benefit becomes permanent, the Community Choice Act offers states financial assistance to reform their long term service and support system to provide services in the most integrated setting.

"Specifically what does this bill do?

1. Provides community-based attendant services and supports ranging from assistance with: activities of daily living (eating, toileting, grooming, dressing, bathing, transferring), instrumental activities of daily living (meal planning and preparation, managing finances, shopping, household chores, phoning, participating in the community), and health-related functions.

2. Includes hands-on assistance, supervision and/or cueing, as well as help to learn, keep and enhance skills to accomplish such activities.

3. Requires services be provided in THE MOST INTEGRATED SETTING appropriate to the needs of the individual.

4. Provides Community-based Attendant Services and Supports that are: based on functional need, rather than diagnosis or age; provided in home or community settings like – school, work, recreation or religious facility; selected, managed and controlled by the consumer of the services; supplemented with backup and emergency attendant services; furnished according to a service plan agreed to by the consumer; and that include voluntary training on selecting, managing and dismissing attendants.

5. Allows consumers to choose among various service delivery models including vouchers, direct cash payments, fiscal agents and agency providers. All models are required to be consumer controlled.

6. For consumers who are not able to direct their own care independently, the Community Choice Act allows for 'individual's representative' to be authorized by the consumer to assist. A representative might be a friend, family member, guardian, or advocate.

7. Allows health-related functions or tasks to be assigned to, delegated to, or performed by unlicensed personal attendants, according to state laws.

8. Covers individuals' transition costs from a nursing facility or ICF-MR to a home setting, for example: rent and utility deposits, bedding, basic kitchen supplies and other necessities required for the transition.

9. Serves individuals with incomes above the current institutional income limitation – if a state chooses to waive this limitation to enhance employment potential.

10. Provides for quality assurance programs which promote consumer control and satisfaction.

11. Provides maintenance of effort requirement so that states can not diminish more enriched programs already being provided.

12. Allows enhanced match (up to 90% Federal funding) for individuals whose costs exceed 150% of average nursing home costs.

13. Between 2007 and 2011, after which the services become permanent, provides enhanced matches (10% more federal funds each) for states which: begin planning activities for changing their long term care systems, and/or include Community-based Attendant Services and Supports in their Medicaid State Plan.

SYSTEMS CHANGE

14. Provides grants for Systems Change Initiatives to help the states transition from current institutionally dominated service systems to ones more focused on community based services and supports, guided by a Consumer Task Force.

15. Calls for national 5 -10 year demonstration project, in 5 states, to enhance coordination of services for individuals dually eligible for Medicaid AND Medicare."

http://www.democraticunderground.com

Community Habilitation /Day Habilitation

Community Habilitation is a service provided for individuals who need day supports and planned activities provided by a companion/aide. This service can be provided to an individual or as part of a group day program.

Day Programs

Programs of planned activities developed for people with severe disabilities who usually are unable to work in a marketplace or supported employment setting. Day programs can be organized educational and activity programs all available on one site to serve a large group of people, or they may be community-based activities where individuals meet in a central location and then are accompanied out into the community for daily activities. Other day programs may be work oriented, or involve individuals in volunteer projects.

Direct Service Professionals

Also called personal care attendants and aides, DSPs work directly with people with disabilities to facilitate activities of daily living, and support what individuals need to enable them to live as optimally in the community as is possible.

www.dspspeak.org/SPEAKWEBSITE.htm

Dreams With Wings

A residential program developed in Louisville, Kentucky to provide apartments and other appropriate housing for individuals with primarily cognitive disabilities. Dreams also offers a day program and other varied programs and activities for their residents and friends of the program.

DSM IV

Diagnostic and Statistical Manual, 4th Edition – American Psychiatric Association's definitive listing of psychiatric diagnostic conditions.

Facilitated Communication

"Facilitated communication . . . is one form of augmentative and alternative communication (AAC) that has been an effective means of expression for some individuals with labels of autism and other developmental disabilities. It entails learning to communicate by typing on a keyboard or pointing at letters, images, or other symbols to represent messages. Facilitated communication involves a combination of physical and emotional support to an individual who has difficulties with speech and with intentional pointing (i.e., unassisted typing).

"The person who provides support is called a facilitator. A facilitator can be a teacher or other professional, a family member or a friend. This support is highly individualized, based on specific needs. Thus it does not look the same from person to person. . . .

"The goal of facilitated communication is for individuals to achieve independent expression, often with a combination of typing and speech."
http://thefci.syr.edu/About_Us.html

Family Broker

A paid or volunteer advocate who acts as a coordinator of services, funding, and futures planning for an individual and their family.

Futures Planning

"Futures planning or person-centered planning has a number of features that distinguish it from service planning:

The focus is on the individual's whole life – not just services, not just a type of service.

The plan is the person's plan – not an agency's.

The people involved in the planning are there at the person's invitation – no agency decides who should or must be involved.

There is an emphasis on involving friends and family in the planning – professionals participate to advise and not control.

The focus is on a vision or a dream for the future, practical ways to get there, and building commitment – not starting from compromises based on what is.

The emphasis is on the person's strengths, gifts, and talents, building on them and supporting the person in areas of individual needs – not a preoccupation with deficits and assessments of 'what's wrong with the person.'

The challenge is how the individual, family, friends, and services (not only services) can work together to achieve the vision.

The person's plan may serve as a focus for discussions about what services should be provided. A service plan may then result.

"Futures planning represents a radical shift. It amplifies the voice of people with disabilities, their families and friends. It looks at capacity in people and communities.

"Futures planning did not ignore disability, it simply shifted the emphasis to a search for capacity in the person, among the person's friends and family, in the person's community, and among service workers. A person's difficulties were not relevant to the process until how the person wants to live was clear. Then it was necessary to imagine and take steps to implement creative answers to this key question, 'What particular assistance do you need because of your specific limitations (not labels) in order to pursue the life that we have envisioned together?'"

Connie Lyle O'Brien, John O'Brien and Beth Mount, "Person-Centered Planning Has Arrived.... Or Has It?" *Mental Retardation*. December 1997.

Graphic Facilitation

Graphic facilitation is a way to use images to organize ideas in a meeting. By using images instead of just notes, the facilitator opens up creative possibilities and ideas not accessible by words alone. Visual learning opens participants to new ways of seeing an issue or situation, allowing for new approaches to problem solving and strategy development.

www.alphachimp.com/tour/tour_gf.html

Group Homes

Supported residences usually for three to eight (sometimes up to sixteen) individuals and round the clock staff to care for their needs and coordinate their activities. May also be a single family home providing services to several individuals.

(Also called board and care home.)

Haldol

Haloperidol is indicated in the management of manifestations of acute and chronic psychosis, including schizophrenia and manic states. It may also be of value in the management of aggressive and agitated behavior in patients with chronic brain syndrome and mental retardation and in the symptomatic control of Gilles de la Tourette's syndrome.

www.mentalhealth.com/drug/p30-h02.html

HCBS

Home and Community Based Services – "1915 (c) waiver – Medicaid home and community-based services waivers that allow states to request waivers of certain federal requirements to allow development of HCBS treatment alternatives to institutional care so long as these alternatives cost no more than it would to provide the same care in an institutional setting."

www.hcbs.org/glossary.php

HCBW

Home and Community Based Waiver. Same as above.

HCFA

"The Health Care Financing Administration (HFCA) was created as a principal operating component of the Department [of Health and Human Services] by the Secretary on March 8, 1977, to combine under one administration the oversight of the Medicare program, the Federal portion of the Medicaid program, and related quality assurance activities. Today, HCFA serves 67 million people, or one in four elderly, disabled, and poor Americans through Medicare and Medicaid. In fiscal year 1993, HCFA will spend an estimated $230 billion to provide health care services."

www.os.dhhs.gov/about/opdivs/hcfa.html

Home Habilitation

"In-home habilitation services include daily living services and related training, e.g., personal assistant services, homemaker services, routine wellness, and community integration services such as skills training, peer support and community integration activities and field experiences."

Housing Authority

Public housing agencies in cities that are mandated to provide decent and affordable housing for low- and moderate-income consumers.

HUD

Housing and Urban Development – HUD is a Federal Agency overseeing all aspects of housing in the U.S. that fall under government regulation, financing, and availability issues.

"HUD's mission is to increase homeownership, support community development and increase access to affordable housing free from discrimination."

www.hud.gov/about/index.cfm

147

ICF-MR Facility

"Intermediate Care Facilities for persons with Mental Retardation. Usually institutional settings serving large groups of individuals. Currently all 50 states have at least one existing ICF-MR facility usually with 15 or more residents. But since the implementation of the current regulations in 1988, there has been a major shift in thinking in the field of developmental disabilities. Emphasis is now on people living in their own homes, controlling their own lives and being an integral part of their home community."

www.cms.hhs.gov/CertificationandComplianc/09_ICFMRs.asp

IDEA

Individuals with Disabilities Education Act – "The Individuals with Disabilities Education Act (IDEA) is a law ensuring services to children with disabilities throughout the nation. IDEA governs how states and public agencies provide early intervention, special education and related services to more than 6.5 million eligible infants, toddlers, children and youth with disabilities.

Infants and toddlers with disabilities (birth-2) and their families receive early intervention services under IDEA Part C. Children and youth (ages 3-21) receive special education and related services under IDEA Part B."

http://idea.ed.gov/

ISP

"The ISP, Individual Support Plan, describes the kind of life that a person wants to live, including their dreams, goals, community activities and experiences that would allow them to achieve their desired outcomes. It reflects the insights gathered through the person-centered planning process."

For a detailed outline for an ISP plan see:

www.tennessee.gov/tenncare/forms/sdwaiverISP7106.pdf

Kentucky Independence Plus

"Kentucky's Independence Plus Program is part of the National Cash & Counseling Demonstration Program which allows Medicaid members who require waiver services to purchase those services differently. The program is a joint effort between the Department of Medicaid Services, the Department for Mental Retardation, and the Division of Aging Services."

arcofky.org/CDO/index.html

Medicaid

Medicaid (Title XIX) is a Federal- and state-funded program of medical assistance to low-income individuals of all ages. There are income eligibility requirements for Medicaid.

Medicaid Waivers

"The Social Security Act authorizes multiple waiver and demonstration authorities to allow states flexibility in operating Medicaid programs. Each authority has a distinct purpose, and distinct requirements

"Section 1115 Research & Demonstration Projects: This section provides the Secretary of Health and Human Services broad authority to approve projects that test policy innovations likely to further the objectives of the Medicaid program.

"Section 1915(b) Managed Care/Freedom of Choice Waivers: This section provides the Secretary authority to grant waivers that allow states to implement managed care delivery systems, or otherwise limit individuals' choice of provider under Medicaid.

Section 1915(c) Home and Community-Based Services Waivers: This section provides the Secretary authority to waive Medicaid provisions in order to allow long-term care services to be delivered in community settings. This program is the Medicaid alternative to providing comprehensive long-term services in institutional settings."

http://www.cms.hhs.gov/MedicaidStWaivProgDemoPGI/

Medical Model

The "medical model" has its strengths in some arenas, particularly those in which there is substantial consensus among humans as to what constitutes a "problem" and such problems reflect situations involving fairly simple cause-effect relationships. In other arenas, of which mental health is a significant example, the "medical model" has clear limitations. Among these are

- an over-reliance on "categories," "ideals," and "objectivity"
- a failure to appreciate the significance of internal experiences
- lack of appreciation for diversity and for the essential role played by individuals in their own evolution
- lack of appreciation for the role of culture in mental health

http://serendip.brynmawr.edu/sci_cult/mentalhealth/models/mentalhealthmodels2.html

Medicare

"Medicare (Title XVIII) Is a Federal health insurance program for persons age 65 and over (and certain disabled persons under age 65). It consists of 2 parts: Part A (hospital insurance) and Part B (optional medical insurance which covers physicians'

149

services and outpatient care in part and which requires beneficiaries to pay a monthly premium)."

http://www.medicare.gov/

Mental Retardation

"Mental retardation is a term used when a person has certain limitations in mental functioning and in skills such as communicating, taking care of him or herself, and social skills. These limitations will cause a child to learn and develop more slowly than a typical child. Children with mental retardation may take longer to learn to speak, walk, and take care of their personal needs such as dressing or eating. They are likely to have trouble learning in school. They will learn, but it will take them longer. There may be some things they cannot learn."

http://www.nichcy.org/pubs/factshe/fs8txt.htm

National Cash and Counseling Demonstration Program-

On May 9, 2002, Secretary Thompson unveiled the Independence Plus initiative in response to Executive Order 13217, in which the Department of Health and Human Services (DHHS) promised to provide states with simplified model waiver and demonstration application templates that would promote person-centered planning and self-directed service options.

Independence Plus is based on the experiences and lessons learned from states that pioneered the philosophy of consumer self-direction. Specifically, two national pilot projects demonstrated the success of these approaches in the 1990s: (a) the Self-Determination project in nineteen (19) states, focused primarily in the Home and Community-Based Services § 1915(c) waivers, and (b) the "Cash and Counseling" project in three (3) states, focused on the § 1115 Demonstrations. These programs afforded service recipients or their families the option to direct the design and delivery of services and supports, avoid unnecessary institutionalization, experience higher levels of satisfaction, and maximize the efficient use of community services and supports.

www.cms.hhs.gov/independenceplus/

Person-Centered Planning

"Person-centered planning is a process-oriented approach to empowering people with disability labels. It focuses on the people and their needs by putting them in charge of defining the direction for their lives, not on the systems that may or may not be available to serve them. This ultimately leads to greater inclusion as valued members of both community and society."

www.ilr.cornell.edu/edi/pcp/

Pervasive Developmental Disorder

"The diagnostic category of pervasive developmental disorders (PDD) refers to a group of disorders characterized by delays in the development of socialization and communication skills. Parents may note symptoms as early as infancy, although the typical age of onset is before 3 years of age. Symptoms may include problems with using and understanding language; difficulty relating to people, objects, and events; unusual play with toys and other objects; difficulty with changes in routine or familiar surroundings, and repetitive body movements or behavior patterns. Autism (a developmental brain disorder characterized by impaired social interaction and communication skills, and a limited range of activities and interests) is the most characteristic and best studied PDD. Other types of PDD include Asperger's Syndrome, Childhood Disintegrative Disorder, and Rett's Syndrome. Children with PDD vary widely in abilities, intelligence, and behaviors. Some children do not speak at all, others speak in limited phrases or conversations, and some have relatively normal language development. Repetitive play skills and limited social skills are generally evident. Unusual responses to sensory information, such as loud noises and lights, are also common."

http://www.ninds.nih.gov/disorders/pdd/pdd.htm

REACH

"Founded in 1987, REACH [Resources for Education, Adaptation, Change & Health] of Louisville is an organization committed to person-centered, family-friendly, community-based, and integrated services. Our program offerings include therapeutic foster care, adult foster care, family support, program planning and evaluation, software application development, statistical and geographic analysis, community planning, and program-oriented consultation."

www.reachoflouisville.com/

Section 8

"The Section 8 Rental Voucher Program increases affordable housing choices for very low-income households by allowing families to choose privately owned rental housing. The public housing authority (PHA) generally pays the landlord the difference between 30 percent of household income and the PHA-determined payment standard – about 80 to 100 percent of the fair market rent (FMR). The rent must be reasonable. The household may choose a unit with a higher rent than the FMR and pay the landlord the difference or choose a lower cost unit and keep the difference."

www.hud.gov/progdesc/voucher.cfm

Seven Counties Services

"Seven Counties' Developmental Services provides an entry into the community's service delivery system for persons with developmental delay or disability, and is the regional planning authority for mental retardation and other developmental disability services.

It is a private, non-profit corporation. By state statute, however, Kentucky's community mental health centers are responsible for comprehensive planning and resource allocation in the areas of mental health, mental retardation and other developmental disabilities, and substance abuse for their regions."

http://www.sevencounties.org/

Sheltered Workshops

"A sheltered workshop is an organization that provides employment opportunities for people with disabilities and/or those from disadvantaged backgrounds, such as ethnic minority groups, the long-term unemployed, and those returning to the workforce after a period of rehabilitation. The word 'sheltered' refers to a protective environment where disadvantaged people can undertake paid meaningful employment in a supportive environment."

www.accessiblesociety.org/topics/economics-employment/shelteredwksps.html

Service Coordinators – Case managers – Support Coordinators

"Service coordinators assist consumers to assess their need for services, arrange and coordinate the services, and monitor the services. Different programs use different terms, including 'case managers,' 'care managers' and 'service brokers.' Case Manager is the term for 'service coordinator' used by the Medicaid Program and some state HCBS programs. In addition to assessing the need for services, arranging and coordinating services, case managers may also approve or 'authorize' payments for home and community based services."

www.bulletinboards.com/v2.cfm?comcode=FLSC
www.sevencounties.org/byf_final_2008.pdf

Small Business Development Center

"The Greater Louisville Small Business Development Center (SBDC) provides training and consulting services to for-profit small business owners as well as entrepreneurs wishing to start a small business. The Greater Louisville SBDC offers personalized consulting that is comprehensive and individualized to meet particular needs."

www.louisvillesmallbiz.org/

Social Role Valorization

"Social Role Valorization (SRV) is the name given to a concept for transacting human relationships and human service, formulated in 1983 by Wolf Wolfensberger, PhD, as the successor to his earlier formulation of the principle of normalization (Lemay, 1995; Wolfensberger, 1972). His most recent (1995) definition of SRV is: "The application of what science can tell us about the enablement, establishment, enhancement, maintenance, and/or defense of valued social roles for people" (Wolfensberger, 1995a)."

From a 1998 article by Joe Osburn, "An Overview of Social Role Valorization Theory, *The International Social Role Valorization Journal/La revue internationale de la Valorisation des roles sociaux,* 3 (1), 7-12.

http://communitygateway.org/text/tutorials/srv.htm

Social Security

"Social Security, in the United States, currently refers to the federal Old-Age, Survivors, and Disability Insurance (OASDI) program.

"The Social Security Act, as amended, includes several social welfare or social insurance programs. The better known programs of the Act are:
- Federal Old-Age, Survivors, and Disability Insurance
- Unemployment Insurance
- Temporary Assistance to Needy Families
- Health Insurance for Aged and Disabled (Medicare)
- Grants to States for Medical Assistance Programs (Medicaid)
- State Children's Health Insurance Program (SCHIP)
- Supplemental Security Income (SSI)"

www.ssa.gov/

SSI, Supplemental Security Income

"A program of support for low-income aged, blind and disabled persons, established by Title XVI of the Social Security Act. SSI replaced state welfare programs for the aged, blind and disabled in 1972, with a federally administered program, paying a monthly basic benefit nationwide of $512 for an individual and $769 for a couple in January 2000. States may supplement this basic benefit amount."

www.ssa.gov/pubs/11000.html

Supports for Community Living

"This is a home and community-based waiver under the Kentucky Medicaid program and was developed for Kentucky residents as an alternative to institutional care for an individual with mental retardation or developmental disabilities. SCL allows an individual to remain in or return to the community. Services include: case management; residential supports; adult day training; supported employment; commu-

153

nity living supports, behavior supports, psychological services; occupational therapy; physical therapy; speech therapy; respite; and specialized medical equipment and supplies."

www.sevencounties.org/mental_retardation_other_developmental_services.htm

Supported Living

"Any Kentuckian with a disability recognized under the Americans with Disabilities Act is eligible to apply for a Hart-Supported Living grant. The program is administered through the Department for Mental Health and Mental Retardation Services, but it is a program for people with all disabilities. You (and your family, friends, and the people who support you) should consider applying for Hart-Supported Living grant if:

You want to live in a home of your choice that is typical of the homes where people without disabilities live.

You want to participate in your community with all members of the community.

You want to decide for yourself what supports and services you need to live in the community.

You want to arrange for and manage your own supports."

http://mhmr.ky.gov/mr/supportedliving.asp

TASH

"TASH is an international membership association leading the way to inclusive communities through research, education, and advocacy. TASH members are people with disabilities, family members, fellow citizens, advocates, and professionals working together to create change and build capacity so that all people, no matter their perceived level of disability, are included in all aspects of society."

Many people want to know what the acronym TASH stands for. Here's a brief history of the organization's names. When TASH was started in 1974, it was called the American Association for the Education of the Severely/Profoundly Handicapped and went by the acronym: AΛESPH. In 1980 the name was changed to The Association for the Severely Handicapped, reflecting TASH's broader mission. The name was changed to The Association for Persons with Severe Handicaps in 1983 but the acronym, TASH, continued to be used. In 1995, the Board voted to maintain the acronym because it was so widely recognized but to stop using the full name of the organization as it didn't reflect current values and directions.

www.tash.org/index.html

www.tash.org/WWA/WWA_what_acronym.html

TIPP

A group home established by Seven Counties Services (then River Region Services) as a residential, therapeutic, and training program for hard-to-serve children and youth with concurrent diagnoses.

Visiting Nurses

"The Visiting Nurse Associations of America (VNAA) is the official national association for not-for-profit, community based home health organizations known as Visiting Nurse Associations (VNAs).

"Visiting Nurse Associations (VNAs) created the profession of home health care more than 100 years ago. They have a united mission to bring compassionate, high-quality and cost-effective home care to individuals in their respective communities."

http://www.vnaa.org/vnaa/g/?h=HTML/AboutVNAA

Wraparound Support

"The wraparound process is a way to improve the lives of consumers who have complex needs. It is not a program or a type of service. The process is used to help communities develop individualized plans of care. The actual individualized plan is developed by a Wraparound Team, the four to ten people who know the consumer best, including the consumer and their family. The team must be no more than half professionals.

"The plan is needs-driven rather than service-driven, although a plan may incorporate existing categorical services if appropriate to the needs of the consumer. The initial plan should be a combination of existing or modified services, newly created services, informal supports, and community resources, and should include a plan for a step-down of formal services."

http://cecp.air.org/wraparound/intro.html

Appendix C

Summaries of minutes of Raymond's group

When Raymond's group talked about what we wanted to include in this book we thought about all the years of minutes that had been collected and filed. Knowing that reading ten years of meeting minutes would be a daunting and dull task, we knew we would not add them in their original form, no matter how graphically interesting they might be. (Using graphic facilitation often left the group with piles of paper maps to summarize into minutes to be sent out and shared. Raymond loved the job of copying and delivering and/mailing the minutes out to members of his group.)

We knew though, that we would have given a king's ransom to have had the records of any other group doing what we were trying to do. It would have been a valuable guide to spark our own creativity and to give us ideas on fresh ways to approach each barrier we encountered on the journey. So we decided to compromise and offer brief summaries of the early years' activities, and more detailed accounts of the later years. A cursory look at these notes could offer the reader some good ideas to test, some snags and errors to avoid, and some laughs at our stumbling and bumbling.

Year One Summary

The Raymond Atherton Futures Planning Support Team first met in October of 1991. The initial goals set, after reviewing Raymond's history up to that point, included:

Determining what skills Raymond has; realizing his and his family's dreams for him; deciding how he can reach into a bigger world; how he can obtain dependable support for his dreams; how he can go into the world on his own, and how his family could get respite and emergency support.

During two meetings in November the team set strategies for meeting these goals. With Raymond's input they decided he first needed new friends, new interests outside the home, and respite support, "Burly people who care." To get new friends, more team members were recruited who knew others who could be sources of information on funding, agency support and community involvement. Thinking he needed help with his walking, the team was even looking into Raymond having a scooter chair, and he went with his sister, Carolyn to try one out at Bigg.

At the December meeting Raymond reported he liked the scooter, and Betty was working on getting doctor approval in order to get one. Raymond's neighbor Phil Coffin was looking into recruiting a Citizen Advocate.

Betty had been working with Lucy Axton to get Raymond's SSI in order so that he would be getting appropriate funding. Tim was looking into provision of funds from the Home and Community Based Waiver of Medicaid to be able to set up paid respite and other support services. Milton began visiting with Raymond out in the community and Raymond was starting to tolerate his meetings a bit better.

Year Two Summary

Thirteen people met in January of '92 and discussed Raymond's bowling and visits to K-Mart and McDonalds. He'd visited his sister Dana at work and spent time with Nancy Brucchieri. He was more trusting and talking and a bit more willing to try new things. Milton pointed out that this needed to be done gradually.

Lucy had organized the SSI problem and showed how a back payment needed to be spent. Community supports such as Citizen Advocacy and a parent support group had not materialized, but Raymond anticipated dinners out with Carolyn and more outings with Milton.

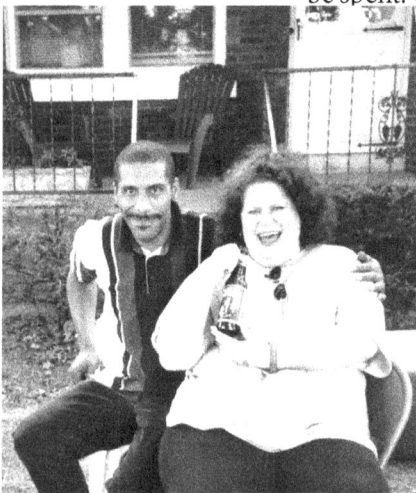

Tony Miles and
Linda McAuliffe.

Six members and Raymond met in February. Raymond's scope continued to broaden with visits with Milton (see Milton's notes in Appendix D), making copies and computer disks, and even playing Nintendo with reluctance. Raymond was attending a Sunday school group with Milton on a fairly regular basis

The group realized that the Home and Community Based Waiver wouldn't work for Raymond's need for respite hours. Recruiting a Citizen Advocate wasn't working, only producing "brick walls." The group was aware that "people resources" need to be able to deal with the unpredictability of Raymond's moods.

April found Raymond going out more with Milton, Tony, and others. He attended a basketball game with Tony. He was doing well at Kinkos helping with copy jobs for the group. Friends were becoming aware of Raymond's sense of humor, as he played jokes on them. Betty learned more about trusts and SSI at a meeting and Hope would update the group on the new Supported Living program.

Nine of the group met in May to share about Raymond's energy level rising, and his attendance at bowling and a field day. He was helping with yard work and painting, and with Denise's move. People in the community are asking about Raymond. He even parted with the last Cola, for Milton.

In June he was going to Kinko's and Target and coping with things like storms and broken copiers with increased patience. Betty described it as Raymond holding up better under family chaos. Hope was looking into a neighborhood grant which would promote opportunities for community friends for people with disabilities

Fall marked Raymond's first positive reaction to a "new meeting." He was disappointed at missing a planned church service. He shopped for a new jacket and went to the Zoo with Tony. Betty felt he'd been "back-treading some," in his reactions to change, but the group felt he had done a lot of new things.

Year Three Summary

January '93. Would Supported Living Funds be forthcoming? Raymond's new experiences increased, including van washing and a job volunteering at Highland Presbyterian Church.

March '93 found big changes in Raymond's situation. With his SSI and Supported Living Funds in place, Raymond was spending (Community Habilitation) time with his friend Jim Schrecker picking up loads for Kentucky Harvest and visiting the Fitness Center to ride the exercise bike and swim. He briefly helped with coffee at Sunday school, and was looking into doing volunteer work at Highland Presbyterian. Things were working more smoothly in new areas for Raymond and Betty actually began to think about getting away for a few days. This was an unheard-of idea two years before.

Raymond and Jim S. made trips to Otter Creek for camping. This was a big step toward being away from home and being confident with some independence. Raymond bought a new sport coat to wear to a benefit concert. He had a haircut with Milton and had his portrait made. His social life was expanding. He had dinner out with Jo Ann Boyle, and Nancy Brucchieri. He went to Kinko's to print and then deliver his group minutes.

In July the family had concerns over Betty's mother's illness. They spoke with Renelle Grubbs, then of Seven Counties Services about possible grief issues for Raymond. Betty felt that two years of positive progress needed some shoring up in the face of a possible big loss in Raymond's life.

The Athertons decided to celebrate all of Raymond's success with his new friends at a fish fry on October 4, Raymond's birthday.

Raymond began visiting an art therapist in November as a way of developing new ways of expressing feelings. The team felt that this might be a way for him to deal with grief more effectively. He kept track of his own appointments and set them with his therapist according to his schedule.

Raymond took less Haldol at Dr. Greenberg's recommendation and the urging of the team. The drowsy side effects were making it hard for him to get through his day.

The team remarked at this time that Raymond was more confident, more relaxed, and better able to state his preferences, likes, and dislikes. This relieved anxiety for him and apparently lessened his outbursts.

At this time Nancy Brucchieri took on the role of family broker, funded by Supported Living dollars.

Raymond, Milton, Nancy and other group members had been looking all three years for a church home for Raymond that would accept him and honor him as a member and provide more people in his life to relate to and connect with in the community. Aside from Raymond's job preparing bulletins for Sunday services, no other church community made a fit for Raymond.

The group joined Raymond for a Christmas get-together. All had a good time.

Year Four Summary

1994 opened with a bang and a big January blizzard. The first meeting was held in February. Raymond's dad had been ill, and Raymond had an accident which landed him in the hospital with a cut hand. With family, and Jim Schrecker's support, that was a survivable situation, but required round-the-clock back-up.

The family had long been looking for a primary care physician that would really work with Raymond. Raymond managed to visit his dad in the hospital, again with Jim Schrecker's support. He also would visit when Jim saw his own doctor in order to develop a comfort level with doctor visits.

Raymond met with Gene Baker, the behavioral psychologist from Seven Counties Services, who expressed amazement at the terrific changes that had occurred for Raymond.

Raymond was getting more involved in using different equipment at the spa and enjoying it. He was improving his bowling scores with Jim.

He attended a religious program at the Convention Center with his family. He was bothered by the darkness and the lights, but he had a new experience and it was pretty good.

Milton was on the Supported Living Council at this time and he made useful recommendations about preparing the SL grant reapplication and funding update due in March.

The team was looking into reading tutoring for Raymond at this time. Contacts were made at U of L and JCC, but the group wasn't successful in making a strong connection with tutors for Raymond. Jim Schrecker felt that Raymond's continuing improvement in communication skills would be supported by a reading tutor.

Despite Carolyn's baby due date, the Fish Fry was held as planned in Betty and Jim's backyard.

The team held a long-range planning meeting in September. In this meeting the group brainstormed on all the possible ways that Raymond could live more independently, and how those ways could be achieved. They included: Fostering, or Family Home Provider; Raymond living in parents' home with live-in supports, while parents move; Raymond having his own place in an apartment, with supports living in; a committed community such as the L'Arche model; or a cooperative housing setting through Seven Counties Residential provision.

Situations which had to be built into any plan were gradual transition, live-in supports, closeness to family, Raymond's choices, and a setting with plenty to do in the vicinity.

With day supports in place, and Raymond's emotional situation improving, the family and the team felt they could begin considering a move with more confidence. Raymond's days were busy with Kentucky Harvest volunteering, the spa, and daily errands.

But still on the drawing board were tutoring issues, church contacts and finding a personal physician.

Team members planned a trip to TASH in Atlanta to talk about Raymond's Futures Team and his progress and circumstances. This was an extremely rough experience for Raymond who found the airplane and the trip away very anxiety-provoking. The trip left Raymond in a difficult place for some time after.

Year Five Summary

Nancy Brucchieri opened the year with a letter to the team. She stressed the importance of the support of each member to the team.

1/18/95

Attached are minutes from our last regular meeting and from our long-range planning session in the fall. My Martin Luther King resolutions (I make mine then instead of New Year's Eve) include trying to do a better job of getting these to you in a timely fashion! I hope that you have continued to feel kept up with things, however, as we usually talk with each other between meetings. I also hope that each of you realize the importance that you bring to the group both with your resources and your friendship. If there is any way that I can make our community work better for you, please do not hesitate to let me know.

We decided not to keep minutes from our brainstorming session at Carolyn's on Jan. 3, 1995. It was a time to talk more in depth together about Raymond's trip to Atlanta, to support Betty as she sees evidence of things not going as well with Raymond, and to see if we could find any other resources to keep the situation from deteriorating further.

Basically, we realized that most of our work/planning has been based on the hope/assumption that Raymond would continue to maintain what had been seen in the past few years. We realize that we also need a contingency plan if that does not happen.

Hope has contacted Herb Lovett [a psychologist from Boston] who is willing to meet with us on March 17 to discuss Raymond's situation and give his insights, etc. He has asked that we obtain some neurological tests prior to his visit. We are currently working on this as well as ways to pay for the visit, etc. Please try to keep as much of this day open as your schedules permit. We will have more details on this to follow.

We are also asking the Supported Living Council for additional money to pay for additional family support to lessen the impact that Raymond's behavior has on his family during this period.

Our next meeting is Wed., Jan. 25, 1995 at Raymond's house. We decided it would be best to include Raymond in this meeting and therefore moved it back to his house rather than at Tim's.

At the January meeting Tim took over from Linda as resource coordinator. Because of Raymond's anxiety since the TASH trip the group requested additional funds from Supported Living to provide some weekend and evening support. Linda explained that in-home-support resources could be used for time outside the home that would support Raymond's family situation since there could be no additional Supported Living funds in this year. The team needs to put efforts into recruiting staff to support Raymond on weekends and in the evenings.

Hope said that Clinton's rental house was coming available since he was buying a home. The group discussed the possibilities of renting a "transitional house" for Raymond. Hope said she would talk to Carolyn Wheeler about a trial lease. (Carolyn is Clinton's guardian and would know the landlord.)

The next meeting found the end of Raymond's spa experiences. The new owner of the spa would not allow Jim to visit as Raymond's friend, insisting on both joining. They stopped going. Raymond was enjoying his art "classes" more and coping with new experiences better.

Linda's crew had not yet found an in-home support person.

Hope had arranged for Dr. Herb Lovett to visit Raymond for a day and offer his opinion on what things could go better for Raymond.

On March 17 Herb Lovett came and began a day with Raymond at 9:00 a.m. They visited for a bit before Tim and Raymond went to breakfast, and after breakfast Herb joined them for their activities around the community. At 11:00 Ray, Nancy and Herb met with Julie for observation of Raymond's work there.

12:00: Hope, Linda, Raymond met at Julie's and went to lunch.

Nancy took Herb to the Athertons' for lunch with family.

1:30 to 4:00: The group met at the Atherton house.

Follow up – No one found a neuro-psychologist to work with Raymond, or who would take Medicaid.

It was decided that alternative housing for Raymond would not be timely now. It would be too much for Betty to take on maintenance of a second home.

Supported Living funds were approved in April. The group recruited for someone to take evening hours with Raymond.

In June the group hired Owen McWilliams. Continuing funding was sought to support this. Tim suggested the group look into an application for Alternate Intermediate Services Program funding (now called Supports for Community Living Waiver through Medicaid).

A neuro-psychologist was found and an appointment set.

Raymond and Owen were doing well. Raymond was having hard afternoons just before Owen would arrive. The group wondered if these were signs that Raymond was getting ready to move on. Jim and Raymond were still together for days. They needed to work on more approaches to community involvement.

Raymond would be evaluated in the fall for facilitated communication.

Betty and Raymond participated in a legislative tour for Supported Living.

Raymond was not selected for an AIS slot, and there was a shortage of Supported Living funds. Group members explored alternative funds.

Dr. Walker, the new Seven Counties MH-MR Psychiatrist, was working well with Raymond.

Raymond and Jim continued looking into new volunteer activities: Kentucky Harvest pick-ups of surplus foods on a regular route; Meals on Wheels delivery. They also looked for a new spa membership.

Raymond tried out facilitated communication with Jayne Miller. That didn't work as hoped. They developed a life book instead to help initiate conversation with Raymond and chronicle his days. Raymond asked to learn how to read a menu.

Betty and Nancy wrote for additional supported living funds to finish the costs for Owen's time. They emphasized that the time spent with Owen helps Raymond develop more skills toward independence and living on his own. Owen and Jim are filling in for Tony's weekend time.

Year Six Summary

Jo Ann Boyle was asked to meet with the group in March to brainstorm. John O'Brien met with the group in February for the same purpose.

Betty and Nancy requested more Supported Living funds to finish the year. They also worked on what funds Raymond would need from Supported Living to live on his own.

The group continued looking for back-up people to work with Raymond and fit into the newer plans of Raymond having his own place.

The planning meeting discussed opportunities for Raymond: new home; more self-control; new friends; new job; better communication; more community participation, etc.

Ideas discussed included a purchased duplex, funding sources for down payments, and ongoing support for rental.

Raymond was accepted into the AIS slot. The group needed to choose a provider. Seven Counties, Community Living, and Options for Individuals were explored. These funds could pay for daily residential care, respite, leisure/recreation, live-in care, day program or community habilitation. A plan would be developed annually with an IHP (ISP) meeting (Individual Habilitation Plan – Individual Support Plan).

By April Raymond was away from home from 9 a.m. to 9 p.m. with Jim or Owen. They worked on volunteer work, social times, shopping, meal preparation skills, etc. Transition times were most difficult for Raymond: leaving home and returning home.

Raymond's medicines were reduced. He would request Haldol when he was stressed and knew it.

Seven Counties would cover funding until the AIS funds were in place. Tim worked on revisions to the AIS application. Supported Living funds were increased to fund Owen's work.

Raymond said artwork relaxed him. He continued to dictate poems expressing his observations and feelings. He set a Fish Fry date.

October – Betty and Milton completed a new Supported Living Budget and met with Donnie Shelton, director of the Supported Living plan.

Seven Counties continued working on approval of Raymond's AIS plan. They planned to have respite providers for Raymond to meet.

Raymond spent a week with Owen's family.

Raymond was evaluated by Dr. Schrodt for Tourettes Syndrome. Dr. Schrodt suggested that he needed better control of seizures. Lamectil is prescribed for mood stability.

Respite was needed for Thanksgiving. The group discussed pros and cons of Raymond living with a family member. The group thought it would be unlikely that AIS funds would support paying family as providers.

Carolyn, Raymond's sister, expressed interest in possible building purchase. The group researched KHC and it is not a possible source for a loan. Section 8 might help with supplemental rental for Raymond

Example of task list

What do we do right now?

Owen can spend extra time with Raymond. Jim also can spend extra time.

PASSPORTS can pay. What's needed is $700 for two weeks (30 extra hours a week)

The request meets the guidelines of the Emergency Respite funds which PASSPORTS has available.

What Next?

Tim will request $700 emergency respite funds first thing in morning.

Jim and Owen will work out schedule for extra hours.

Linda will work on letter to Supported Living Council regarding additional funds.

Hope will call Larry Kimberlain regarding the possible availability of start-up funds to help Raymond get set up in an apartment.

Betty and Nancy will look for apartment.

Linda will follow up with Betty regarding the decision of the Community Living Board.

Betty will meet with Cindy Bayes to discuss Seven Counties Services as a potential AIS provider.

Betty will talk with Becca Krall re: a good word to Community Living Board.

Milton will call David Block re: the possibility of Options being AIS provider for Raymond.

Betty will follow up with getting Raymond a new physical.

Tim will schedule a psychological evaluation for Raymond with SCS.

Year Seven Summary

The family and group had continuing concerns over balancing Raymond's medications, and doctors.

Seven Counties Behavior Specialist Jenny Mathis would develop a behavior plan for Raymond as required under the AIS (SCL) funding.

The group continued to discuss possible apartments and how to fund housing and a roommate. Would AIS funds apply? Family Home Provider?

Nancy and Betty completed the Section 8 housing application.

Raymond and Betty hosted a fish dinner for the Ash Wednesday, February meeting.

Minutes excerpt from Feb. 12 – to illustrate funding issues.

The meeting began with discussion of supported living budget.

"We must let Mr.Shelton know if we are going to have any unspent money. Betty will look into cost of purchasing workers comp benefits for Owen, as Mr.Shelton reminded her that Raymond is ultimately responsible for damages if a contract worker doesn't carry the insurance. We are only about $1,225 behind in budget at this point due to time that Owen took off when Grace was born, and from less costly workers comp for Nancy and Jim than had been budgeted. Any money that is not spent for worker's comp we will ask to have available as start-up money for Raymond's apartment. We need to confirm that this will not jeopardize our receiving our full allotted amount next year, which we will continue to need.

"There are several issues that we need to clarify with Cindy Bayes before the next meeting. Hope will arrange a meeting with her. Our goal by the March meeting is to have the ground work laid for moving ahead with beginning to look for an apt. for Raymond, to be able to make a decision about Raymond's relationship with a psychiatrist, and to be clear about upcoming changes in Raymond's income sources vs. continued AIS/MR eligibility."

The March meeting was therefore very important.

The group was still looking for new respite providers. The group asked Lucy Axton if extra funding sources for services would affect Raymond's SSI/SSDI income limits, or how any paid work would affect the limits and by how much. They also checked if it would be a problem for the Supported Living money to go through his checking account.

Nancy, Betty. and Raymond wanted to interview employment providers for possible jobs since Raymond expressed an interest in doing more work like his church job.

JUNE 1997

The group was still working with family to support sorting out medications.

Community Employment committed to working with Raymond around jobs. Raymond met with Linda Irvin at Vocational Rehabilitation for evaluation. Owen expressed interest in a job development position, but some concern was expressed about possible confusion of roles.

The group wanted to find a Community Resource Developer to help plan with Raymond to create a meaningful day for him. They needed to recruit more people around Raymond for supports through AIS.

Linda began facilitating meetings. Nancy stepped back due to job changes. Jim Schrecker left his role as day Community Habilitation worker.

AUGUST 1997

Raymond's day ended up being more broken up. Cliff would spend a short time with him in mornings, but didn't stay very long in the job.

OCTOBER 1997

Cindy Bayes looked at Seven Counties for Community Planning support, and a new Case Manager. She researched whether group members could be providers.

Options would only serve Raymond as AIS pass through, not residential or case management.

Raymond needed two or three support people each day.

DECEMBER 1997

John, Vonda, and Jason were recruited to be new day supports. John proposed days with a "main event" each day for Raymond. Group thinks about this approach.

The group was still looking for a provider for neuro-psychological testing recommended by Herb Lovett. Previous attempts didn't work out.

Year Eight Summary

JANUARY 1998

Sally Shaikun became Raymond's new job coach from Community Employment. Raymond's family was still trying to connect with an appropriate neurologist and psychiatrist.

The group began rethinking possible residential options.

Raymond thought Owen's new house was excellent. The group talked about what a tentative schedule might look like in a new place for Raymond.

Residential Providers were polled by letter to see if they could provide services. Since they all said no, the group could apply for Supported Living Funds to act as residential provider for Raymond.

APRIL 1998

Ray was acting upset over his dad's being ill. He was spending some day time out with John and briefly with Jo Anna. Group was still looking for keys; discussing further consultation.

Need expressed for on-call behavioral support. Linda, Milton, Nancy and Betty will develop Supported Living Application. The group felt a need to move on residential options.

JUNE 1998

Raymond's father died in May. Raymond was distressed but handled things fairly well.

Raymond worked at the church with Sally. Betty set a weekly schedule with Raymond so that he knew daily what to expect.

Gerald and the group developed an ad to recruit people to "life-share" with Raymond. Owen took on recruiting tasks as well as house management.

JULY 1998

SSI said that Raymond must pay back $399 per month in order to keep the SCL. (AIS) funds.

Carolyn and Syd purchased a duplex. Raymond began collecting household goods. Raymond, Carolyn, Syd, and Betty started remodeling the new house. Betty submitted an application for Section 8.

Raymond's group to do list and meeting reminder

1. Betty and Rocky will attend Section 8 meeting on 11/17/98.
2. Betty will see if Owen will facilitate Raymond and Jason spending time to-

gether in order to determine if they are a good match for roommates.

3. Milton will contact Hope about possibly co-sponsoring Wade Hitzing's visit. (This visit may lead to some consultation on Ray's behalf.)

4. Betty will coordinate in setting up a meeting with Karole Duran, OT.

5. Linda will continue to seek respite providers through CAKY /KIPDA.

6. Betty will follow up with David/Owen to make sure that Donovan is meeting all requirements for the funding sources.

7. Betty, Milton, Nancy will meet to revise supported living grant as necessary. Next meeting, Tues. 12/8/98. Holiday gathering.

Year Nine Summary

What is the Matrix of Support around Raymond Atherton?

AIS funds for home care?

Weekdays, 9 to 10 a.m. there is an in-home training need. Currently no provider. Pay requirement, $10 per hour.

AIS Supported, employment.

Community Employment; Recreation/Leisure: Hours needed from 10 a.m., to 5 p.m.

Job coaching and social/leisure time: Each could vary during this time period, depending on job availability. At least 2 different people should be involved with Ray to avoid burnout and reduce stress for all. Also roles could be clarified between work and fun. Ideally, no one person would work with Raymond for more than 4 hours at a time, preferably less. Pay req. $12 -$15 per/hr.

Support out-of-home, from 5 to 9 p.m. This is currently being provided by Owen and Julie McWilliams and will continue. Pay req. $10.

Respite needs: Sat. 10-6 p.m. Providers Owen and Julie $10 per/hour.

Four overnights per month no current providers; pay $10 per hour at $100 per night.

At times two people might be needed to work with Raymond at one time due to possible behavioral crises.

JANUARY 1999

Raymond's house was ready to furnish, remodeling complete.

Group worked on ways to start new staff out with Raymond. There was emphasis on modeling from previous and current staff and family he was comfortable with like Owen, Pat. and Gerald. Careful transitions would be necessary for staff. They should get to know Raymond and he get to know them gradually.

The group identified a continued need for a Community Resource Developer. Group members would each ask specific contacts.

Carolyn Wheeler began to facilitate meetings.

Revisions were needed in Supported Living funding.

FEBRUARY 1999

Raymond got a housing voucher from Section 8, with $350 available to apply to monthly rent. Carolyn arranged for the necessary inspection.

Supported Living approved emergency back-up funds and other requisitions in the revisions to the application.

Owen's family would live downstairs – alternate resident, Gerald.

The group looked at roommate recruitment. Each member made contacts. Hope and Owen worked on a recruitment flyer. All of the group members posted ads or flyers.

APRIL 1999

Owen and Julie moved into the duplex. Raymond spent evenings there, and would go upstairs to spend time in his apartment. Owen coordinated Raymond's schedule.

Furniture was bought before the grant cycle ended.

Raymond liked showing his apartment to visitors. He would stay there when he felt ready.

The new Supported Living Application was submitted.

Still no Community Resource Developer was recruited. Work group decided to share tasks, support Pat and make connections.

Discussion held about Raymond's anxieties. Grief over Jim Atherton's death. Fears of impending move.

The group asked Julie McWilliams to spend some day time with Raymond to relieve Pat.

MAY 1999

Hope moved to Wisconsin.

Rhonda was recruited as new Community Resource Developer – Gwen became new Support Coordinator through Seven Counties.

The small work group would hold a meeting to develop Raymond's day. Forty hours could be paid for by SCL. Two people plus Julie McWilliams. would be recruited and scheduled. All members needed to make an effort to make new contacts.

Understanding the funding "lay of the land."

Supports for Community Living waiver program:

Options for Individuals is "provider agency" for community habilitation (days in week)

Seven Counties Services - Support Coordination, Gwen Harbuck

Supported Living:

Community Resources development - Rhonda Henning

Household Manager/scheduler/ back up - Owen McWilliams

Apartment mate stipend.

Advertisements developed for group to distribute and find venues for.

AD: Caring person needed as housemate for 32-year-old St. Matthews area gentleman; looking for patient, confident, flexible live-in person; free rent and monthly stipend for assistance and household help.

AD: Confident, flexible, part-time day companion and community contact to spend planned, productive days with 32-year-old gentleman; competitive pay; must have driver's license and reliable car.

JUNE 1999

Raymond moved in June 1 with Tony as roommate.

The McWilliams moved out at end of June. Gerald moved in downstairs.

Raymond spent his day time hours with Todd and with Pat.

Supported Living funds were granted for 2000. The Supported Living Council was concerned about any duplication of funds for services.

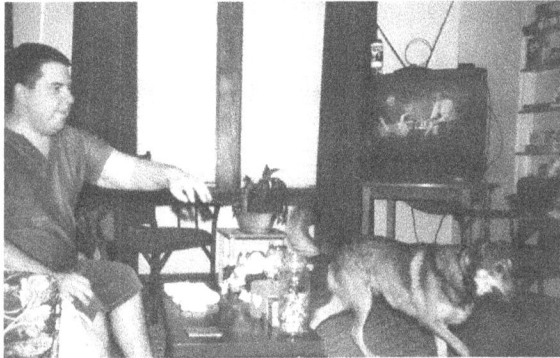

Raymond at home playing with Gerald's dog.

Raymond enjoyed having visitors come to see his home. He still needed more supports for his day. A special meeting was set for June 14 to plan for his day.

Fish Fry, Aug. 21.

NOVEMBER 1999

A new roommate was recruited, Bryan, a student.

Raymond was having difficulty adjusting to new seizure medications. It left him groggy.

Pat worked with Raymond at Frulatti's. Raymond was paid for his work.

Since Jenny Matheis left, Gwen prepared a behavior plan for Raymond.

Milton and Betty looked over the Supported Living plan to assure that there was no duplication of funding for services.

Year Ten Summary

JANUARY 2000

Bryan and his dogs will move in, in February.

Supported Living funding paid for: Household manager – Gerald; Roommate – Bryan; Recruiter – Becky; Workman's Compensation, Group meeting facilitation, and Accounting services.

Lee Bobzien took Gwen's place as support coordinator. Julie Cole was asked to record the history of the group, so other futures teams can use the information.

A meeting to continue planning Raymond's days would be held Feb. 1.

FEBRUARY 2000

Raymond and Bryan were getting along, plus the dogs.

Raymond was looking for a health club. The Y and the Crescent Hill Bubble Pool allowed a supporter along without charge.

Raymond continued working at Frulatti's and church three mornings a week.

The group decided to discontinue the behavior support plan.

They looked for funds to install safety lights in the halls and stairways.

MARCH 2000

Pat became very ill.

Becky needed to recruit for a Community Habilitation supporter.

Group recruited for back-up and respite help for when Betty would go on vacation in June.

Linda wrote a letter showing no duplication of funds for services between SCL funds and funds for the Supported Living Plan

MAY 2000

Celebrate!

1. Raymond lived in his apartment for almost a year.

2. Betty sustained the Section 8 learning curve with great endurance and perseverance.

3. Raymond has been doing the bulletins for over seven years.

4. Raymond really liked his job at Frulatti's

5. The Atherton family's commitment, tenacity, and resilience had been really inspirational in the light of the challenges.

6. Raymond rolled with the changes of people.

7. Gerald and Bryan were really the keys to making his apartment Raymond's home.

8. Fixing up the house helped Raymond to grow "roots" and identify with the apartment as his own.

9. Team effort helped the family to be willing not to fear the unknown.

10. There were fewer problems than anticipated

New things – Raymond did a great job with the Easter Bulletins. Cheryl from CAKY was spending 3 to 4 hours a day with Raymond. The group was looking for another day person through Community Living.

The Supported Living Application was sent in.

Betty's vacation was postponed till July.

Looked for respite workers from KY Opportunities.

Day plan group met May 16.

JUNE 2000

Additional requested funds from Supported Living not approved. The original allocation will require cuts to make it work. Could SCL funds fill the gap? Group efforts were made to see if funds could maintain Raymond's situation.

Ky. Opportunities did not accept Raymond as a respite client.

Nancy looked for Community Employment support for the Frulatti's job. Lee and Carolyn asked Options for employment support.

Occupational Therapy evaluation was recommended to improve Raymond's independence in his apartment.

Pat was at Mt. Holly Nursing Home. Raymond and Betty visited weekly.

Recruitment funding ended June 30.

June 2000 funding

Supported Living budget will cut out every thing except the positions related to the apartment.

Supported Living   Supports for Community Living
        with cuts, short $2668

Apartment Mate   100%
        Cannot be FHP unless lease in provider's name.
        If lease is not in Raymond's name he would lose Sect. 8 certificate.

Household Coordinator   100%
Cannot be staffed residence as Raymond couldn't pay family member.
That also would require staff notes, specialized training.
He couldn't bill community living supports for a day person, because that benefit
        is designed for three-people residences.

Facilitator for Circle meetings	From 100% to 0
Recruitment	From 100% to 0
Respite	100% CAKY /KIPDA
Community Habilitation	100% Options for Individuals.
Community Living Supports	100% Options
Support Coordination	100% 7Cos

Carolyn W. wrote a follow-up letter to the Regional Supported Living Council asking for support for staffing Raymond's apartment, and asking for reconsideration of the requested $2688. Linda wrote a letter explaining why the SCL waiver funding can't pay for Raymond's apartment staff-related needs.

Continued push by all of the group to recruit for Community Habilitation Day coverage, with David Block through Options; Seven Counties; other respite and community living organizations; Community Employment.

Lee will amend Raymond's ISP to include the Occupational Therapy evaluation.

OCTOBER 2000

Bryan moved away.

Gerald developed a flyer to recruit a roommate. Milton pulled together a day staff ad. Lee asked CAKY/KIPDA for help with respite, and in recruiting a Community Habilitation person.

Alex spent three mornings a week with Raymond. Raymond continued to enjoy his job at the church.

1. Lee got a copy of Individual Support Plan out to everyone.

2. Gerald took flyers and met with Seminaries, local churches, U of L Psych Dept. JCC Human Services, U of L Autism Center.

3. Gerald asked Alex if he knew of interested roommates.

4. Everyone on team considered recruitment possibilities.

JANUARY 2001 - Minutes outline.

1. Alex and Ray spend time from 8 to 11:30 Tues., Wed., Thurs.

2. Deer Park Assoc. newsletter will print Ray's roommate notice in March issue.

3. Highland Pres. included flyer in their bulletin, which Raymond folds.

4. Pastor of Springdale put flyer in bulletin and forwarded it out to a number of people.

5. Bellarmine U. put notice in e-mail system and housing dept. Spalding U. will include flyer in housing information.

6. Betty accomplished the Section 8 re-certification in one visit!

7. Not much response to flyers. Not suitable responders.

8. Gwen Harbuck suggested these criteria for recruiter:

    a. knows a lot of people, is well connected.

    b. Solid values

Group will all recruit recruiters. Linda will ask Jenifer Frommeyer, Lee will ask Cathy Saliga. Milton will help Betty include recruiter and future planner as line items for Supported Living funds.

Meeting 9/24/01

Attendees: Linda, Raymond, Julie, Jennie, Gerald, Betty, Carolyn S., Milton, Lee, Sarah, Nancy, Jason & Carolyn W.

What's Happened

1. Fish Fry a great success. Ray stayed out the whole time (4 to 10). (See Chapter 1.)

2. Today marks the 10th anniversary of Ray's futures planning group meetings. Group began in 9/91. Much has been accomplished.

3. Ray has a greater sense of ownership of apartment.

4. Ray enjoys routine, and trying new activities.

5. Recruitment by Nancy Brown not productive to date.

6. Ray working longer than usual at Highland Pres. A larger # of bulletins to put together (post 9/11/01).

7. Gerald and family members have done a remarkable job, as has Raymond, in keeping the situation together despite not having a roommate.

8. Raymond enjoys visiting Lee at her office and bringing her a special treat. Enjoys deliveries.

What Next?

1. Milton to run ad in Southeast Christian Outlook.

2. Denise will run off 100 flyers.

3. Betty will contact pastoral leadership at three neighborhood churches across street.

4. Nancy will contact Presbyterian Center.

5. Julie C. will contact Autism Training Center.

6. Gerald will explore Greater Louisville Website for possibilities.

7. Gerald will explore Insight regarding Community Bulletin Board for advertising.

8. Jason will post flyers at Spalding.

Regarding employment

1. Lee will determine billing mechanisms through Community Living Supports, Community Habilitation and Supported Employment through the SCL waiver for this purpose.

2. Betty will check with Ruth at Highland Pres. regarding other churches where Raymond might assist with bulletins or mailings.

3. Milt will contact Linda Irvin re: Raymond's status with DVR.

4. Milt will brainstorm with Sarah re: Raymond's day.

5. Places for Sarah to contact for possible volunteer activities.

> a. local churches
> b. United Way
> c. Deer Park Neighborhood
> d. St. Matthews Area Ministries.
> e. Dare to Care
> f. Kentucky Harvest.

Next meeting Nov. 1.

Meeting 11/1/01

Attendees: Raymond, Betty, Barry, Jennie, Nancy, Lee, Linda, Milton, Sarah, Gerald, Carolyn S., Julie C., Carolyn W.

What's Happened

1. Raymond is carrying on more conversations and enjoys interacting with people in apts. on Nanz Ave.

2. Recruitment efforts for a roommate by Nancy Brown now productive. Suggest she look at local churches.

3. Raymond has been working longer than usual at Highland Pres. There are a greater number of bulletins to prepare. He does 50% himself.

6. Raymond is following a routine in his apt without having someone to remind him.

7. Julie contacted U of L placement, Autism Center. No response.

9. Jason placed flyers at Spalding.

10. Milton put ad in Southeast Outlook.

11. Nancy contacted Presbyterian Church.USA.

12. Milt spoke with Linda Irvin/DVR – to reopen Raymond's case.

13. Raymond is making choices when he is out shopping.

What's next?

Nancy will contact Amy Hewitt for ideas.

Lee will talk with Mattingly Education Center, connections with volunteers.

Julie asks at Community Living and Council On Mental Retardation, Sr. Debbie Kern at DaySpring, Catholic Employment and Catholic Charities, and Autism Training Center.

Barry will check with Ann Jirkovsky at Bellarmine U.

Betty will talk with grade-school friends at reunion.

Employment possibilities.

Next meeting Dec. 13, '01

Meeting 12/13/01

Attendees:

Barry, Linda Irvin, Lee, Milton, Jennie, Betty, Nancy, Raymond, Sarah, Julie C., Carolyn W.

What's Happened

1. Ray will play Santa at Nanz apartments.

2. Joel Taylor, possible roommate, teaches at Fern Creek.

3. Nancy spoke with Louanne Goldsby at JCC; got 4 contacts, student newsletter, job board, human services program, disability services. Nancy tried to reach Amy Hewitt.

4. Barry spoke with Ann at Bellarmine.

5. Julie spoke with publicity manager at Presbyterian Center, Spalding. Corie delivered fliers at U of L. No response from Autism Center.

6. Lee called LDS church.

7. Betty thanked Nancy Brown.

Work-related ideas

1. Barry, Milton and Linda discussed possibility of Raymond owning own business.

2. D.D. Council might have start-up funds.

3. Milton in touch with SBA re: assistance.

4. Raymond's Vending Service: business plan, two or three machines, Uniform, Hire assistant/driver, Pepsi machines ideal.

Issues to consider

Maintenance, Locations (Seven Counties, Beauty Shop, Pepsi Dist., new businesses, Highland Pres.

Security, storage of items, traffic, liability insurance, publicity, accounting services.

Resources:

Developmental Disabilties Council for start-up cost.

SBA business plan

DVR - Fawn Vending Machine

Next?

Milton and Barry develop business plan.

Jennie check out beauty shop.

Barry check out Highland Pres. & Pepsi.

Betty ask Linda J, re son's experience.

Nancy explore possibility of small candy machines.

Next meeting 1/15/02.

Meeting 1/15/02

Sarah Tackett, Linda McAuliffe, Carolyn Wheeler, Lee Bobzien, Carolyn Stansbury, Gerald Atherson, Betty, Raymond, Julie Cole, Nancy Brucchieri, Vonda Vanderhorst and Becca Krall.

Vonda and Becca came to do scrutiny of SCL and SL programs as they work together in Raymond's life.

Gerald is finalizing recruitment of Alex's friend Shawn. Supported Living can pay part of a year. Gerald is working on dividing up the week to use the money effectively. The residential trainer position is split between Gerald and the roommate. Becca says the grant was at 50% in December. Gerald feels new recruit needs to have probation period before complete pay is given.

Vonda says to reapply 4/1 for next fiscal year at increased funds level. Auditors looked at all recipients of SCL and SL. Services cannot be duplicated, but SL can pay for approved non SCL supports. Vonda doesn't see Ray getting service duplication but that will be reviewed. The support he gets for residential is not available through Supports for Community Living, which only supports staffed residences. SL encourages people to live in their own homes and supports that concept.

There are 1900 people on a waiting list for this; people are trying to get services to as many people as possible. Carolyn says that there is a need to understand services person by person, not to exclude anyone from one program or another.

Milton and Barry will meet with Small Business Association to develop a business plan for Ray's potential vending service. Gerald could place machines in repair businesses. He could get several letters of intent from these businesses for machine placement. They cost $250 apiece. (Betty's niece Linda has two for price of shipping. Realized $25 a week from her collections.)

Need a police check on potential roommate. Gerald said he'd find a Net.com to do it on line, and he'll tell roommate, "You have to have insurance on your vehicle at all times and have a vehicle in working order."

Ray had a good Christmas and delivered a lot of cookies. Betty: "I credit this to Sarah. She planned a list with him and that took the tension out of it. He enjoyed the Christmas party at Dreams on Nanz. He played Santa. He demonstrated his, 'HO, HO, HO.' It was impressive."

End of the minutes summaries of Raymond's Futures Planning Group.

Appendix D

Milton Tyree's notes

The following are edited notes from Milton Tyree from 1992-93, when he first began to spend community time with Raymond. These notes provide a glimpse into the trial and error mode that Milton, Jim Schrecker, Owen McWilliams, and others used when spending good times with Raymond. We include them to share the ideas for things "to do" and how Milton particularly did those things with Raymond as they got to know each other.

4/6/92

Raymond and I went to the main branch of the library today around 2:00. He was anxious to go when I arrived – so afternoon hours do not seem to be an issue with Raymond. (Actually, Raymond was in very good spirits – teased me about the tie I had on at his PFP meeting last week, etc.)

Before entering the library, I explained to Raymond that people inside were reading so it would be necessary for us to talk quietly inside. He had been talking pretty loudly. However, once inside he very consciously lowered his voice. Once again Raymond was willing to accept guidance about what is "socially acceptable."

He helped me search the data base for a couple of books which were not available. He hit the return key after I entered the needed info. Then we went to the desk to get a replacement for my library card, which I lost last week. He seemed to get a little bit tired with all of the walking, but he never complained. When I asked if he was tired, he said, "No."

I asked if he would like to run some business errands with me on Friday, and Raymond said, "Call me." I said that I will call him on Friday morning to set a time.

4/10/92

Raymond and I went to Kinko's to make copies and to my post office. He was helpful as usual. It stormed when we were gone and Betty had been concerned that this would bother Raymond. Actually, it did not seem to bother him at all.

I told Raymond that I needed to get some presentation materials ready on Monday afternoon. I asked if he wanted to help. He said, "Yes; call me."

4/13/92

Once again, Raymond and I went to Kinko's. However, today Raymond did assist with a new copier task of making transparencies. I hand-fed the film and placed the originals on the glass. Raymond placed the originals on top of the completed transparencies, closed the lid and waited for me to tell him to hit the start button. He did very well. We need to find other things to do. I suggested this to Raymond and he said, "Yeh." The time is right. We agreed that I will call him Thursday afternoon regarding his assistance with errands on either Thursday afternoon or Friday morning. . . .

4/23/92

I went to Kinko's (sans Raymond). One of the clerks asked me, "Where's your friend?" I told him that I was out on my own today. The clerk said, "Well tell him that I said Hi."

4/29/92

Once again Raymond and I did the Kinko's routine. He was in an exceptionally good mood – quite talkative about many topics: He asked me about my weekend; he told me about his "vacation"; he told me about his sister Denise's new house; he teased me about a number of things including not wearing a tie, about not getting an answer at his house when he and Betty were staying at the Red Roof Inn last week (during home construction); about taking wrong turns, etc. Also, Raymond struck up a conversation with a couple who were waiting to use our Xerox machine at Kinko's. He also asked the clerk at Kinko's, "Where are the girls?" in reference to the woman manager who is usually there.

On the down side, Raymond's grandmother (Betty's mother) is critically ill. However, Betty said that she wanted to keep Raymond's schedule as routine as possible. I said that I could use some help this Friday afternoon. Raymond said, "Fine." . . .

5/6/92

Raymond copied and mailed two letters with me today. He did very well with the tasks, but he seemed less comfortable with the clerks when he paid for copies and mail. Essentially, Raymond "rapid-fired" questions such as "Where is your car? – Where is your wife/husband? – Are you busy?"

Raymond was talking louder than usual, not in a conversational sort of way. Perhaps "being in charge" of paying and getting the receipts is increasing Raymond's anxiety to the extent that he feels less comfortable with people. At any rate, I need to pay extra attention to preparing Raymond for these "interactions," and for now take a more active role in the interaction. (Mainly because his style today caused some degree of negative attention from the clerks, and others standing nearby.) . . .

5/12/92

Raymond went with me to get money from a Quest machine and to pick up some office supplies from the Office Depot. He was in excellent spirits. The only new venture was operation of the Quest machine. I directed Raymond (pretty much hand-over-hand) on inserting the card and operating the buttons. Despite the extent of my intervention, Raymond seemed to enjoy the activity. . . .

5/21/92

Raymond and I went to Kinko's, Target, and the Post Office together. I backed off a bit on Raymond's responsibilities with clerks, and I suggested to Raymond that he not inquire about the whereabouts of clerks' cars. This resulted in a more relaxed time (and Raymond did not ask about cars). When we returned Betty said that Raymond had been increasingly reluctant to go out since returning from Golden Field Days, which she reported as a very positive experience where Raymond shot basketballs for the first time in years. I did not notice any difference in Raymond's interest in engagement with me or others today. We agreed that I will call Raymond on Wednesday to see if he wants to go on more errands with me. Raymond said that he would want to go....

5/29/92

I picked up Raymond at his sister Carolyn's house today since his house was being painted and he preferred not to be there. We went to Kinko's to copy a report. Two interesting points from today: 1. Before we went inside Kinko's, I reminded Raymond not to ask people about their cars or spouses since these questions may confuse people. I suggested the he talk about other topics instead. He did so. 2. It was raining very hard today and the roof on my car was leaking pretty bad – right on the top of Raymond. However, he took this right in stride, did not become upset at all and even thought that it was funny....

6/11/92

I called Kelly McClendon (St. Paul's Methodist Church) to follow up on my visit to the "Tower" group (newsletter) and to see if there are other groups within the church where people are Raymond's age. (The Tower group had not worked out, due to crowding and group demeanor.) ... I was told there were three Sunday School classes ... which may provide ways for Raymond to get to know others.... Kelly suggested the Seekers class which consists of single and married people in their 20s and 30s. 5 to 10 people attend. Also this class meets in a casual setting in a house next door which he felt may be inviting for Raymond.

I called Raymond and asked him if he wanted to run some errands with me today. No one was home, so I left a message on their tape, AND Raymond called me back and left a message on my tape saying that he was available to help me. When I saw Raymond later today, I told him that I appreciated the message and he seemed quite proud of his accomplishment....

I discussed my conversation with Kelly McClendon with Raymond and Betty. We agreed that I will attend the Seekers Class as soon as possible to get to know the members. If it "seems right," I'll introduce Raymond to this class. Betty felt that the Sunday class would be the best place for Raymond to meet the members rather than a social event. I could see Raymond attending a class with me with the understanding that the primary purpose (initially) would be an introduction so we may leave early.

Raymond was quite open to pursuing this process. We had discussed it in the car prior to talking with Betty. . . .

6/15/92

Raymond and I went to Kinko's to make copies. My primary purpose for asking Raymond to help me today had to do with attire. I knew that I would be wearing a tie and I had called Raymond a couple of days ago to tell him so and see if he would be willing to do the same. He didn't, but the occasion did bring up the topic of Raymond getting some long pants to wear. (This is something that Betty has been talking to Raymond about doing. She said that he only wears short pants during the summer and sweat pants during the winter.) I told Raymond that if he would get some long pants, then we could go more places and meet more people. He smiled and said, "Yes." Betty said that they would go shopping on Wednesday. This is truly a significant step in Raymond being seen in a more positive way and especially regarding his pending visits to St. Paul's Methodist. . . .

Also noteworthy today, was Raymond's conversation with the clerks at Kinko's – not cars or spouses. Instead he said, "Good morning – are you busy, and bye." I said that I will have some work to do on Thursday. Raymond said, "Call me."

6/27/92

Raymond and I went to the Bardstown Rd. Kinko's and to the main Post Office.

Raymond did very well "socially" in both places without any reminders from me. He joked with an employee of Kinko's who was leaving with her bike. "Don't run over me." Also he took care of giving two of Betty's packages to the postal clerk and paying for the packages. I was standing beside him, but he handled the situation very well and did not seem anxious.

Betty commented before we left that the summer heat was affecting Raymond's energy level. This seemed to be true as Raymond was walking very slowly. I asked if the heat made him tired and he said, "Yes."

For the first time I saw Raymond have what Betty calls a "Haldol freeze" and what Raymond calls "Playing dead."

This happened after we returned to his house. Betty said if this occurs when we are out that Raymond can understand directions and walk with support, to get home, etc.

I understand that the same thing happened earlier this week at Hope's house. Betty said that this is an unexpected side effect of the Haldol, which Raymond has been taking for seven or eight years. She hopes that the psychiatrist will see fit to reduce the Haldol, since Raymond has also been taking lithium since last summer and she largely credits the lithium with helping Raymond control his anxiety.

6/28/92

I attended the Seekers class. The teacher asked me to talk to the group briefly about Raymond and my goals for him through the class. The group was very welcoming and indicated that they would be glad for Raymond to attend.

After class Angie Leet and I tentatively set up a time for her to meet Raymond for Wed. the 1st at 6:30. I said that I will see Raymond on Tuesday and we agreed that I will call her to confirm....

7/1/92

Raymond, Betty, Angie Leet, and I went to McDonalds for a Coke. Raymond and Betty were quite comfortable with Angie. Angie and I asked Raymond to attend the Seekers class this Sunday. He seemed to be interested, yet was not willing to make a firm commitment. We agreed that I will call him at 9:00 on Sunday morning to see if he would like to go with me. We drove by the church and the house where the class meets on the way back home. I think that Raymond is intrigued with the idea of attending the Seekers class.

7/3/92

... [After checking out the St. Anthony's Soup Kitchen as a possible place for Raymond to volunteer by handing out bread in the lunch line] Dana and I went to McDonald's to review our perceptions of this place for Raymond. We determined that the job of passing out bread would be one which Raymond would enjoy. However, we felt that additional visits would be in order to get a better idea of the pace of this job if it was determined to proceed with developing this as a place for Raymond to go. We felt that the location was not very convenient in terms of Raymond's home. Also, we discussed the disadvantage of Raymond not meeting people from his own neighborhood. The desirability for Raymond meeting others with whom he may form a relationship to do other things was also doubtful here, since the people who volunteer are mostly of retirement age. Also the people coming here to eat were people similar to Raymond in that their lives had of late been characterized by rejection and failure. On a related note we determined that it would be most desirable for Raymond and the people coming to the soup kitchen to have opportunities for relationships with people who are perceived by society in a positive way. ... Dana and I will share our analysis with the group at the next PFP meeting.

7/5/92

Raymond did go with me to the Seeker's class today! He wore new clothes, khaki pants, a polo shirt and sports shoes and looked really sharp. He stayed for about twenty-five minutes and generally seemed to be very comfortable. Raymond was quite conscious of wanting to "fit in." He spoke quietly to me from time to time when he had a question about what was happening. Susan and Angie followed us out and told Raymond that they hope he returns. He indicated that he would. I explained that I will be out of town for possibly the next four weekends. Angie asked Raymond if he would like to ride with her when I am out of town. He said, "Call me." It was a very positive experience.

7/19/92

I ended up being in town after all and Raymond went to the Seekers class again with me. He asked to leave after about a half hour. Susan then asked if she could show Raymond around the church. Raymond agreed. They were gone for about 15 minutes. Both seemed to enjoy the occasion....

8/12/92

I attended Raymond's PFP meeting. We agreed that I will do the following before the next meeting: 1. Visit the Deer Park Baptist Church senior citizen luncheon in the company of Max. Hope will make initial contacts and let me know when I should contact Max for the purpose of looking into luncheon help roles for Raymond.... 2. Follow up with Angie about the idea of Raymond initiating pre- or post-Sunday school outings with fellow class members. 3. Follow up on information regarding Raymond assisting volunteers who deliver meals for Highland Community Ministries. 4. Follow up with Carol Long regarding a role for Raymond assisting at St. Andrew's Episcopal Church.

Also discussed was preparing information about the types of services which Raymond is now receiving. (What are Raymond's service needs? What would we call this type of service? Who provides it? How much does it cost?) Plans of this sort are needed to insure that Raymond continues to have services available following the end of REACH....

8/28/92

I introduced Raymond to Carol Long, the secretary at St. Andrew's Episcopal Church. She asked Raymond to help her copy some flyers. Carol instructed Raymond in the operation of the copier and I assisted Raymond with the instruction on different "runs" of the flyer. I added a step which Raymond has not done before – the recording of marks on a piece of paper so that we could track the number of total copies. By the time the work was completed, Raymond knew how to start a run of copies and record the run. Next time we will work on positioning of paper – done today by Carol. We stayed for approximately twenty to thirty minutes. Most important Raymond and Carol seemed to "hit it off." I will be working out of town next week, so the three of us agreed that Raymond will next assist Carol on September 10th....

9/6/92

Raymond and I went to the Seekers class. He looked great in his new clothes and was anxious to go to the class. Raymond said that he had gone to the class last week with Angie. The group today was small and Raymond was very conversational – he has some new topics to discuss. He asked me about my trip to Bowling Green when we were in the car, and at class he asked Angie about her recent trip. We stayed for the entire class this time. A first for me and Raymond. Although I believe that he has done this before without me.

183

Raymond is becoming more flexible and listening to the wishes of others. For example, today he asked me one time if we could leave class with about 15 minutes left. I said that I would like to stay, and he said, "OK." Also, Betty told me today that Tony asked Raymond if he wanted to go to the zoo last week as they were returning from a planned trip to Value City. She said that Raymond said, "No," but when Tony said that he really wanted to go to the zoo, Raymond agreed and that he had a good time....

9/10/92

I called Carol today to confirm Raymond assisting her. She said that she did not have work for Raymond to do today because she thought that I had arranged for Raymond to work on Friday the 11th. Due to other commitments, I cannot give Raymond a ride tomorrow. However, next week we will be able to start a regular Tuesday trip to St. Andrew's so that Raymond can assist Carol with preparing the church's weekly newsletter.

I called Raymond to explain the mix-up and said that I would like to come see him anyway. When I arrived Raymond asked about Carol, but seemed OK with the change in plans. He looked really sharp – had on new gray slacks and a navy polo shirt. We went to McDonalds' for a late breakfast. After we sat down Raymond decided that he wanted a Coke. He said, "I'll wait here." I suggested, "Why don't you go get your Coke and I'll wait here?"

I gave him a dollar; he went to the counter and asked, "Do you have a small Coke?" He paid, came back to the table and seemed pleased with his accomplishment....

9/13/92

When I called Raymond this morning, he asked if we were going to have donuts at the Seeker's class. We decided to buy a dozen on the way to class- a decision appreciated by all. Raymond wore a new sports coat today – very sharp! We do need to concentrate again on topics of conversation other than "Where's your car?" Other class members are confused by the question. Raymond and I can probably think about other things to talk about on the way over.

9/22/92

Today was Raymond's first day to assist Carol with the newsletter. He used the copier, folding machine and paper cutter and worked for approximately one hour. I am still assisting Raymond with setting up the copies (setting number and positioning the paper.) he hits the start button and hands the completed work to Carol. This was our first day with the paper cutter and the folding machine. On the folding machine, we work as a team. I do the first part and Raymond finishes the job. Basically I feed the newsletters and Raymond catches the completed letters and places them in the order folded in a box. When using the paper cutter, I aligned the paper and Raymond cut and restacked the paper in order. Raymond was very attentive to stacking the papers right side up. He needed his attention called to the potential danger of the blade on the cutter.

Carol seems to genuinely appreciate Raymond and his assistance....

10/6/92

Today was the day that Raymond and I had agreed that he would get his hair cut by Laura at the Chopping Block.... Raymond was unsure of going out to get his hair cut, since Betty has cut his hair for some time now.... He asked me to accompany him after I introduced him to Laura. Raymond did not especially like having his hair washed before it was cut, but he did not complain at the time. When Laura was done, Raymond said, "I don't want you to shampoo my hair." Generally Raymond seemed OK although not as relaxed as in other new situations that we have tried. He talked to Laura and Karen throughout.

At one point, Raymond yelled, "NO!" I was somewhat taken by surprise since I have not heard Raymond say "no" in this way for months. However, the response in the shop was interesting. No one seemed to be startled. Rather Karen calmly said, "I think that he is trying to scare us." Then Raymond smiled and said, "No, I am sorry." Laura and Karen said, "That's OK." And that was the end of it.

After we were finished, Raymond was noticeably proud of this accomplishment. I think that he will want to return....

10/11/92

Raymond and I returned to the Seekers class at St. Paul's. The whole mood of Raymond's involvement in the class is gradually becoming more spontaneous and relaxed. Raymond's timing of questions is more relaxed and well thought-out. For example today he tended to leave more time for people to respond and he asked questions such as, "How was your weekend?"... Also class members' involvement with Raymond seems more natural and less forced as time goes on. Additionally, today the class ran over and Raymond did not once ask, "Are we going to be done?" Perhaps that explains why the class went overtime....

10/20/92

I called St. Andrew's to speak with Carol to confirm Raymond assisting with the newsletter. I asked for Carol and was told that, "She no longer works here." I explained the purpose of my call to the current receptionist, Jane. She explained that Carol retired from the position last spring and was merely filling in until a new permanent receptionist could be hired. She suggested that I wait until the new hiring to pursue Raymond's continuing with his newsletter responsibilities.

I went to Raymond's house anyway and explained the situation to Raymond and Betty. We will need to find something else for Raymond to do on a regular basis – something that he can look forward to doing and find purposeful....

I told Raymond that I needed to go to Sears to get a part for my lawnmower and

I said that I would like for him to go with me. We went to Sears, but Raymond was quite disappointed about Carol leaving St. Andrew's. He asked about her many times and apparently did not understand how she could just disappear....

10/26/92

I attended Raymond's PFP meeting. I reported the information about the possible van ride to church and about Wesley night (A regular Wednesday dinner at St. Paul's). Raymond and other group members felt that these were good avenues to pursue. Also, I will follow up about the status of the receptionist position at St. Andrew's.

Betty is concerned that Raymond is "regressing" – getting louder at home, feeling more insecure about leaving. While I have not seen this with Raymond, I certainly believe that Betty's concerns are legitimate. These concerns provide all the more need for Raymond to find engagement in activities with others where he can be successful and find meaning....

11/3/92

Raymond and I got together today. He told me that he had gone to the Seekers class with Jennifer. Betty added that Raymond invited Jennifer in to show her his key chain collection after they returned from the class.

Raymond went with me to get my car serviced. We needed to wait for about thirty minutes. Initially, Raymond did not seem too comfortable with this, asking, "Are they going to be done?" But after a few explanations about the work to be done, approximate time frames, and how we would be informed when the car was finished, Raymond was OK with the wait.

11/5/92

Raymond accompanied me to select a birthday gift for Vicky. He teased me about Vicky finding her present in the trunk of my car before the big day.

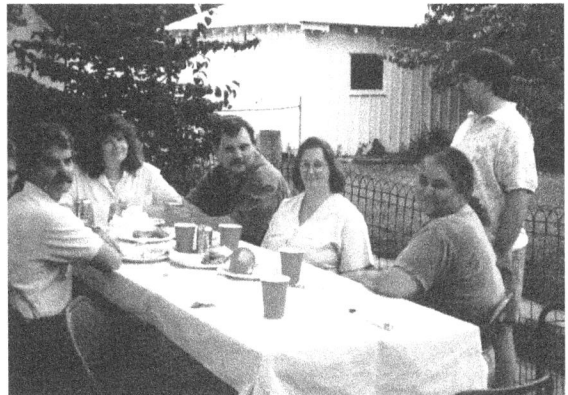

From left, Milton Tyree, Carol and Tim Estes, Vicky Tyree, Nancy Bruschieri, and Raymond.

11/10/92

Raymond had agreed last week to help me rake leaves at my house today. But, alas, it was raining. He accompanied me on some errands to Target and the VW place instead. Actually, he seemed quite relieved with the rain-out.

I told Raymond that I was going to be checking out the Wesley night dinner tomorrow to see if there is something there that he might like to assist with. He said that this is fine.

11/12/92

I talked to Nancy about her visit to the Deer Park Community luncheon. Too bad that some aspects of this dinner cannot be combined with the Wesley night (which Milton had found not having the best opportunities for Raymond's involvement).

Here food is served. However all are older people and the majority are women.

There is a possibility for Raymond to assist with meal delivery. This is typically done in a pair of people who volunteer to do the work together. Therefore, it was suggested that Raymond could do this if there were someone with whom Raymond would like to pair up.

Nancy has also checked with the Highland Presbyterian Church regarding need for office assistance. They are in the process of securing some new equipment so that they will be typesetting and duplicating bulletins in-house. Nancy will check back in about a month to see if there is a way that Raymond may want to be involved....

11/15/92

Raymond and I went to the Seekers class together. He had to miss last week because I was working and a ride could not be found. However, it is significant that Jennifer had helped him seek a ride.

Today, Raymond came out to the car before class, and I dropped him off after class. We have done one part of this before, but this was the first time that I have not gone into Raymond's house at some point during the course of one of our ventures. Raymond seems to like this approach – I believe that he appreciates the independence. I like it because this feels more balanced to me.

Raymond and I also talked about my visit to Wesley night. I said that I thought that he may want to attend, but that I did not believe that they needed any new volunteers at this time. I promised to follow up on other opportunities.

11/16/92

I called Betty to update her on the Wesley Night. She agreed with my analysis. We talked about Raymond's involvement with Jim (Schrecker) This is very exciting and provides a whole new dimension for Raymond's involvement.

11/20/92

Raymond and I got together this afternoon. We went to the Ford garage to pick up a part and then we were going to make copies. However, since today was an unseasonably warm day and since my car was filthy, I asked Raymond if he would help me wash my car. At first he was interested, but as we approached my house he became hesitant. I said that if he did not want to help after we got started that he could watch, but that I thought he would enjoy it. Also I said that I would pay him for helping me.

I washed and Raymond rinsed off the soap. He caught on very quickly, twisting on and off the hose, etc. And he did enjoy the work, and knowing that he was doing well. I paid him $5.00 which he seemed to like....

11/22/92

Raymond and I went to the Seekers class. On the way in Raymond got frustrated with me because I made a suggestion about a suitable way of conduct in the class. He yelled, "NO!" We talked about this some before and after class. I explained that I was not getting down on him, but I wanted to offer a suggestion which would help him get to know people. I said that I wanted to apologize if I had hurt his feelings. Raymond seemed OK with this and he heeded my suggestion during class.

On the drive home I asked Raymond if he would like to attend church sometime after class. He said yes and suggested next Sunday. Raymond and I discussed this with Betty. I suggested that I drive again next week to give up some flexibility with our attending of church functions....

11/24/92

I took Raymond to get his hair cut. He wanted to go, but seemed a little anxious about the endeavor. On the way I suggested that Laura could spray his hair with a water-bottle to wet it instead of washing it. After we arrived he asked her to do this. He and Laura invited me to join them. I sat in a nearby chair, but did not talk much. Raymond was quite talkative, asking Laura about her Thanksgiving plans. He was talking a bit on the loud side which called to him some degree of attention. The shop was quite crowded.

At one point Raymond yelled, "NO!" I did not pick up on his reason for the frustration. This got everyone's attention. But Laura asked him if he was OK. He said yes and they proceeded....

Raymond was very pleased when finished. Next time I will encourage him to be patient and to resist yelling NO. I really think that Raymond is comfortable with Laura to tell her of his frustration in a better way. I do not want Raymond to be known as the one who yells no....

12/16/92

Nancy and I discussed her following-up on several potential roles for Raymond: 1. Coming to Nancy's house on a monthly basis to assist with assembly of a newsletter for one of Nancy's organizations; 2. Rechecking the status of Raymond assisting with the newsletter at her church; 3. Checking with a contact which she just secured at the Bellarmine U. Music Department regarding Raymond passing out programs; 4. Checking with Baptist East Hospital re: volunteers who pass out magazines and/or Cokes. When her father was in the hospital for surgery Nancy noted that these tasks may be done by pairs of volunteers....

12/20/92

...I thanked Raymond for the Christmas card which he sent earlier this week. He seemed quite pleased with this acknowledgement. Betty later told me that this is the first year that Raymond has agreed to assist with preparing Christmas cards. And not only did he agree but he wanted to send out cards. Certainly that is a positive sort of indicator for an expanding world....

12/30/92

Raymond accompanied me to Kinko's to make copies. Raymond did something today which he has not done before: When I asked him to set the number of copies (5) and he hesitated, I started to guide his finger to the correct number. However, when I did this Raymond had gently pulled his hand away from me without saying anything, and then proceeded to set the number correctly without assistance. He continued to set the numbers on request for other pages to be copied. I think that his initiative is wonderful.

12/31/92

Jim Schrecker, Nancy and I met to discuss our current individual activities with Raymond, share ideas about ways that Raymond might spend his time, coordinate the development of new activities, and think who would be able to support Raymond in his new activities.

Jim explained that he is spending time with Raymond 3 days a week from 10-12 and this schedule will soon be increased to 4 days. Jim spends time with Raymond in different activities outside of the house. He is experienced in providing instruction in functional skills in natural environments. I explained that I typically see Raymond briefly 2 times a week: Once to attend the Seekers class at St. Paul's and another time where Raymond accompanies me on miscellaneous errands.

The three of us agree that it would be good for Raymond to have a regularly scheduled activity such as a volunteer job where he could have a sense of purposefulness and routine. We discussed that given time and work in a fitting sort of volunteer position, Raymond could become interested in some sort of employment for pay in the future. Some desirable characteristics include: a. people who would have an interest in Raymond and his success; b. a volunteer job which is structured so that two volunteers share the job so as to increase the likelihood that Raymond may volunteer there without our presence, develop more balanced relationships within the volunteer role, etc.; c. a job where Raymond had a change of environments such as assisting with meals-on-wheels deliveries; d. consideration for Raymond's low energy level, including flexible scheduling; and e. tasks which involve Raymond giving something to someone.

Nancy described the contacts which she is currently seeking for Raymond. (See notes 12/16.) Additionally, I explained that I had spoken with Hope about the meals-on-wheels opportunity which would be available for Raymond if we could help him arrange for a co-volunteer. Hope said that she could place an ad in the Deer Park neighborhood newsletter seeking such a person. We all agreed that this may be a good opportunity which could lend itself to Raymond establishing a balanced working relationship with another volunteer. On a similar note, Jim will check with Kentucky Harvest to see if a similar opportunity may exist there.

…Jim is available to do this during his currently scheduled hours. Nancy and I can also be available to assist as our previously scheduled commitments will allow. Also, we discussed that Nancy and I may be better equipped to help with intermittent stuff such as handing out concert programs with Raymond and Jim may be more able to arrange regularly scheduled time for the routine responsibilities.

12/31/92b

First the good news. Raymond wore a tie to the Boar's Head Festival. He looked great!

Now for the disappointing part (at least for me). Raymond declined to stay for the performance. He and Vicky went inside to get seats while I parked the car – since it was raining. In retrospect, it may have been better for me to have accompanied Raymond inside since we know each other better.

Anyway, I joined Raymond and Vicky. Raymond seemed tense. He began asking me questions about the lights, "Are they going to turn that one out too?" And he was beginning to talk just loud enough to attract the attention of others. I asked if he was OK and he said yes. I said that the play would really be fun and I suggested that he try to relax. Raymond responded to this with, "NO!!" (which reverberated quite well through the church, but didn't really cause a problem.) We sat for a while and Raymond wanted to know when we would leave. I asked Raymond if he would like to sit closer to the back so that we could leave early if he wanted to. He said yes, but then when we reached the back of the church he did not want to stay. He wanted to go home.

I went inside with Raymond briefly to explain to Betty that he decided that he did not want to go. I am very disappointed that this did not work out – a little frustrated with myself for not doing a better job of planning and a little frustrated with Raymond for not trying harder.

1/3/93

Today when I picked Raymond up to go to the Seekers class, he thanked me for taking him to church (The Festival), a gesture which I truly appreciated.

The Seekers class was surrounded with confusion today. As usual, I dropped Raymond off just outside the building while I parked the car. This has the advantage of Raymond and I arriving at different times so that other class members have an occasion to see us independent from each other. For this reason, I intentionally take my time parking the car and coming in. However, today this procedure caused me to unintentionally abandon Raymond. Because when I arrived at the class,, I found a note canceling the class for today, and there was not sign of Raymond. On the positive side, Raymond had been resourceful in locating Garrison in the church next door. They were coming back over to the classroom to look for me when we met. Garrison apologized for the mix up and said that he thought that all class members had been notified of the class' cancellation. He invited us to join another class which he was attending today. But I decided to decline the offer. While Raymond was not showing any signs of being upset, he was showing signs of beginning a "Haldol freeze." I apologized to Raymond for leaving him in the lurch, but I told him that he had handled the situation very well. (This may not have been so negative overall since Raymond did accomplish finding Garrison; however, I would not ever arrange for such a new experience without having backup for things not working out.)

When we returned to Raymond's house I told Jim and Betty how well Raymond had done. While Raymond was changing, Betty and I discussed some of the week's events. She said that it was quite possible that today's stress about not knowing where to go had caused the "freeze" symptoms.

Regarding the Festival, Betty said that Raymond seemed to feel bad about not staying, but he told her, "I hated it." He could not tell her why. I suggested that it was probably an overload of new people and situations. He may not know specifically why he was not comfortable. I told Betty that I had been quite disappointed that he did not stay, yet I feel that Raymond is generally trying very hard, as evidenced today. Betty agreed and said that she thinks he is backsliding, but that he is fighting it. . . .

1/22/93

Today Raymond said that he wanted me to wait up front while he got his hair cut. On the way I suggested that if he felt himself getting tense, that he tell Laura this instead of saying, "NO!"

Well, this seemed to work OK. I heard Raymond tell Laura this once as they were walking toward the back, "I'm tense." So I know that he was trying. I'm pretty sure that I also heard one "No!" as I waited up front. Most important thought is Raymond's effort, interested in going places on his own, and a developing sense of what it is to be an adult.

Also, he is getting to know a bunch of new people who treat him in an accepting and respectful manner, and his hair looks good. . . .

1/24/93

Today the Seekers continued planning with Sherry regarding changes in class structure. Raymond really likes Sherry. He is quite attentive and periodically smiles and contributes to the planning. For instance today when Sherry said that we will complete writing the goals and objectives for the class next week Raymond said, "Wonderful!" Everyone agreed with Raymond on this point.

It is really hard to describe, but Raymond really looked good in class today. He was relaxed, attentive, involved and sitting comfortably on the couch. When we broke into work groups he went with the change very naturally. And he was not in my planning group. . . .

2/1/93

Raymond and I went together on a string of errands. I think that it is significant that today I called Raymond to ask if he would like to go with me to help and we set up a time to meet. Raymond did not ask for his mother to get on the phone and he was ready and waiting when I arrived.

Also Raymond went to Seekers yesterday with Angie.

2/2/93

I called Michael about Raymond assisting with programs at the 3/7 concert.... The job which I believe would work best for Raymond involves taking people's tickets and handing them a program.

Raymond and I stand on either side of a door to take up tickets and hand out programs. This way Raymond can watch me to see what to do, and he can be near someone who he knows well. Also I can assist in directing people with reserved seats to the usher needed.

I will arrange in advance for a backup usher to take Raymond's place should he decide that this is too much and wants to go home....

2/7/93

Raymond and I went to Seekers. A new teacher has been assigned for the month. The class culture has changed in its reorganization stage. Although this is hard to describe, I felt a sort of awkwardness today regarding Raymond's involvement. Raymond was talking more than usual ... which seemed disruptive to the class process which is more formal.

It occurs to me that Raymond has an opportunity to talk and share with other class members before and after class, yet he has no involvement during the class during the content/study portion. Therefore, if he says anything during the class, it is likely to be off subject and therefore disruptive. I want to talk to other class members and think of a way to make this better, e.g., give Raymond a responsibility/role for the class such as taking the collection (new leadership roles have been formalized as part of the class reorganization). Also it seems that questions relevant to the issue being studied could be constructed for and directed to Raymond.

1/8/93

I called Lynell, the Seekers class coordinator. She was very supportive of such ideas. She suggested that members take time at the beginning of the next class to discuss ways to enhance Raymond's involvement, and ways that the class may run smoother for everyone.... She said when I first started talking tonight that she was afraid that I was going to suggest Raymond not coming to class – she wants him to continue to be a part....

2/14/93

Today was a mixed day of encouragement and frustration. I initially went to Seekers without Raymond as planned. The coordinator and I discussed ... ways to involve Raymond in the class discussion and find a "class role" for him as well. I said that I could not attend class the next week but we decided that I would discuss some of the content area with Raymond prior to next week and then call her with questions/issues for Raymond's involvement

I also explained to the class that Raymond wants to fit in and that while he has learned a lot about being a member of a group, that he still needs additional information about this. I said then that members should be comfortable in giving Raymond respectful guidance in this direction. For example, if Raymond engages an individual member in a conversation at a time that is disruptive to the flow of the class, that he may be redirected by saying something like, "We all need to listen to John now, OK?" (Garrison had taken this tack in the past with Raymond, but others have not.)

I picked Raymond up and he was very pleased to join the class. However, when Jeanie attempted such a (quiet and respectful redirection) Raymond yelled, "No!" The class went on, but Jeanie was duly startled and "froze." Also Raymond did not apologize as he has done in the past (e.g., when getting his hair cut).

At the time, I felt frustrated and actually quite angry with Raymond. Jeanie was trying to be helpful. Raymond knows her well and the group as a whole is being quite accommodating and patient with him. His unwillingness to reciprocate seemed very selfish to me.

A little later I left the room after Raymond had left to use the restroom. I told him that I felt it would be a good idea to apologize to Jeanie after class, because she was trying to be helpful and he scared her. Raymond indicated that he would apologize and did so (with my reminder) following class.

2/15/93

I called Lynell and suggested that it may be best to try the changes in Raymond's participation when I am present so that I can (at least initially) facilitate his involvement as needed. I added that I do want Raymond to be able to attend the class without my presence, but given the number of recent changes a conservative approach may be best. Lynell said that this sounded fine and that she looked forward to Raymond's increased involvement in class.

2/17/93

Raymond and I went to McDonald's for coffee/Coke and to talk. I told Raymond about the changes which had been discussed for his Seekers class involvement and he was very receptive. Then we talked about ways to get to know people in the class. I said that I knew that he was welcomed as a class member, and I encouraged him to be patient with members – even if they said something to him that he did not like – for instance Jeanie's comment to him last week. I told Raymond that I was really proud of all of the new stuff he is trying and doing, and that part of being out in the world is handling situations that do not go the way we want. I said that I know that Jeanie did not want to hurt his feelings and that he did not want to scare her. I told Raymond that sometimes when I find myself in a tense situation that I take a deep breath and release it and that this helps.

I was very impressed with Raymond's attentiveness while I was saying all of this. I believe that he understood everything that I said and I also think that he will try to be more patient with others who inadvertently hurt his feelings. He even tried taking a deep breath and agreed to try this the next time that he fells like yelling "NO" in Seekers.

I told Raymond that my parents will be visiting this weekend so I will not be going to Seekers. I said, too, that since we are going to be changing his involvement that it may be good for both of us to be there initially. He seemed OK with this. Betty seemed to think that this would be a good strategy. I told Raymond that I will call him Monday. This was a very good experience for me and I hope for Raymond.

2/24/93

Raymond and I went to McDonald's to talk about Seekers class this week and plan for his participation in the content portion of the class. Raymond was interested in talking about class, but did not want to specifically talk about the content. We talked again about the need for patience with people in class and changes in format. He seems OK with this.

2/28/93

Raymond and I went to Seekers. The class had a relaxed feel. Raymond was patient with others and I believe that he is thinking about the stuff that we have been talking about....

3/3/93

Raymond helped me with the Kinko's thing. We talked about his KY Harvest work that he is doing with Jim. Raymond is very pleased with his work here. Also when we drove by Nancy's church where he helps with bulletins, he talked about this and said that he had seen Linda who works at the church.

We will get together Friday to meet with Michael about ushering at the benefit concert this Sunday....

3/7/93

Raymond and I went to Seekers. We have a new teacher for 6 weeks, Bob. Bob and Raymond seemed to hit it off just fine. Also Wes redirected Raymond once when Raymond had gotten off the topic at hand. ("Let's look at the materials now, OK?") And Raymond did fine with the suggestion.

Raymond decided not to go to the concert (to hand out programs) later in the evening. He was exceedingly tense about going. When I suggested that he did not have to go, he was ready to get out of it. Betty believes that this may be due to the time of day. Raymond is used to going places during the day and staying home in the evening.

At any rate, I went to the concert and I saw one of Raymond's class members, Linda. She said that she and Melody had come up with some "role" ideas for Raymond within the class: 1. Post weekly class announcements on the bulletin board and remind members to look at changes on the board; 2. Help set up coffee before class and help clean up after class; 3. Count the class collection money. (I told Linda that I do not think that Raymond has the skills to count the collection at this time, but that this is something to discuss and investigate with Raymond.) Of course the significant part here is that class members took the initiative to come up with ways to involve Raymond.

Also, Betty came to the concert later and I introduced her to Linda. Linda told Betty how much she liked having Raymond as a member of the class and that she hoped that Raymond would want to start participating in class social functions. This of course was quite sincere, and I believe that Betty was pleased.

3/12/93

Raymond and I got together at McDonald's. I told him about my conversation with Linda and he was very open to trying these roles. We will go to Seekers together on Sunday.

3/14/93

Raymond was ready to make the coffee. He recalled our discussion and reminded me on the way to Seekers. But when we got there another member had already made it. Raymond still put up an announcement on the board and we washed out the coffee pot after class. He enjoyed the responsibilities. Today's class felt very comfortable.

3/21/93

Raymond wore a tie to Seeker's today.

3/24/93

I attended Raymond's PFP meeting. Raymond's life is becoming a busy one. Our only special events prior to the next meeting will be the Seekers brunch on Palm Sunday and a haircut with Laura next week.

3/28/93

At Seekers the class discussed next week's brunch which is to follow class. Raymond was repeatedly asked if he was coming and he consistently answered, "Yes." Raymond and I agreed to bring muffins to the brunch.

3/31/93

I gave Raymond a ride to get his hair cut today. On the way we talked about things that he could do to help out Laura such as asking her to attend his meeting and not saying, "NO!" He followed through with both of these suggestions. They said they were both pleased, and so was I.

End of available notes made by Milton Tyree on visits with Raymond from April 4, 1992 to March 31, 1993. At this time Milton was making these visits as part of REACH.

Appendix E

Edited notes from art therapy sessions – 1994 through 1997

6/30/94

Raymond came in and sat with his Pepsi and talked for a bit. Then sensing he had sat long enough, we got up to do a marker drawing on the shelf. The initial image was a canoe. He surrounded it with water, rocks and a canoe-sized fish. He added green and yellow trees and bushes and was satisfied. He went back to add more green at the bottom. He was pleased with the large image and went right on chatting about it. He said he'd had enough art, but felt that Nancy had a few things she wanted to talk about. Nancy laughed right out, since she knew this was an opener for further conversation. We talked about vacation and summer plans, till Ray announced a bathroom stop. Nancy then said he'd been improving in decision-making and conversation in general. After a bit more chat, he decided it was time to go.

7/21/94

Watercolors. He was tickled to direct me in some of the work. When we do it again I may be more directive to make a more pleasing product. We returned to finish the collage. He again maintained interest. The only time he got even a tiny bit agitated was when I left the room to get a plate palette. The only occasion for "outbursts." We had some great jokes and laughs.

9/8/94

After working on a word list I suggested he take it home and practice each one daily. Then he said he'd had enough, but he had more time. "Nancy wants to talk to you about art work," he said several times.

9/22/94

Ray came in and we chatted extensively over meals and needs and what we've done and intend to do. Ray really enjoys our talks so I am concentrating on them a bit. I may learn more about what he is thinking. We did a word review. He was thrilled when he'd get one right. "WOOOOW," he'd whoop and clap his hands. He managed to connect all the words with limited prompts and it was clear to Nancy and me that more had been learned than just word recognition.

On his way out Ray wanted to say good bye to Leigh, a manager in the offices downstairs. "What's your girl's name?" he said to me like an average visiting executive waving his arm at her desk.

10/10/94

Ray's mom is out of town. (Connect with schedule from Hope.) Nancy said that he was a bit hyper since his mom was out of town, but that he's been doing quite well during her absence. This is a big breakthrough for Ray.

His second drawing was a pumpkin which proliferated into 10. He asked if I had seen them all at the Kroger. He added his name in a lighter orange and volunteered that he really liked orange. "Do You?"

He wrote a poem,

> Dear Mom
> I love you
> I love you
> I will come to get you
> I will come to get you.
> You want to go?
> I will pick you up at the airport.
> You want to go?

11/3/94

When Ray saw the abstract map of the US he recognized that it had letters on it. When I asked what a map was for he said, "Vacation." Nancy prompted with a story about an anticipated trip to TASH in Atlanta. He was excited about that.

12/2/94

Ray came in in high spirits, asking his usual array of questions. During his bathroom break Nancy asked, from the group, if they should work on lessening his persistent questions. I said only gradually since they were his primary means for connecting. If he could be encouraged to ask questions for new information, that would be better than repetitions. He gets good feedback from others' answers, but is not quite secure in giving answers himself.

He laughed right out at starting new words, and enjoyed that the first word was "Happy."

Nancy asked if he should come more often. I said it was up to him, but let it still be a treat and not become routine. (Still concerns about TASH trip.)

1/5/95

Ray in good humor, even though he was locked out of the front door.

He did 40 word recognitions with only 4 prompts. We did finger paints, but mostly by proxy. He loved making prints. Tried to elicit feelings about the "bad" days since TASH, but he was more interested in talking about the TVs he got for Christmas.

2/23/95

Finger paint, third try. Ray actually touched the paint by moving it around with a paper towel.

3/18/95

Herb Lovett's visit. Ray used a sponge for the finger paint.

4/5/95

Raymond bounced in elated and ready to work. He laughed at every word. He liked horn which he identified as trumpet, and then as instrument. He knows so much more than he can let out.

4/19/95

Betty and Nancy. Betty expressed a wish for a parent support group. This never came about. She was looking in vain for doctors to take on Raymond. "Easter was awful. It's not worth having. My energy sinks out the bottom of my feet and I get dysfunctional." Raymond was jolly and fine at art, but at home this had been a dark and painful winter, since the TASH visit. Herb and the "apartment talk" – has that caused him to cycle up? His worst time of day was from 1 to 5. Jim is doing mornings, and with further hours approved takes him a few hours on Sunday.

5/16/95

Ray not his jolliest self. Used outbursts to deal with new ideas in collage. He is painting the whole paper now, whereas when he started he did little shapes around the page. He made three bathroom visits and then said, "Wow, I feel better," after the third visit. He calmed down a bit then too.

6/8/95

Introduced idea of partnering a painting. This was uncomfortable for Ray. He suggested that Nancy and I demonstrate after thinking about it in a bathroom break. He actually supported Nancy's arm as she painted. That didn't upset him.

6/28/95

A fine mood, outgoing and comfortable. I wonder if facilitated communication could work for him since he cannot seem to track words longer than 4 or 5 letters. On the second word project which was things in a house he enjoyed it, saying "This is fun" twice, and "I love you" once. He was concerned about a storm outside but relieved that it stopped when he left. He noticed the noisy fluorescent light, and [was] fascinated by the intermittent air conditioner. On leaving he said "I live here, and I live at Owen's, too." He had recently started spending afternoons and early evenings at Owen's.

7/19/95

Ray had to "go" really when he arrived. He was concerned with a spot on his pants after his urgent need to go. This made for some need to shout during the session. Three free drawings. Graphic development age three or so. Circles and verticals but no encephalopods or other facial gestalt.

8/15/95

Ray came in a good frame, but Nancy said he'd had a couple of bad days, often disrupting his Mom making calls. We had small letter words, and I was hurrying through them. This may have caused some outbursts. I asked him what was going on for him. He didn't share. Ray did ask to end after first project, but I encouraged more, and he did a facial gestalt puzzle. More than any since the first "monkey" but a GD age of only 3 or 4 won't help him with reading.

8/29/95

Ray came in pale, shaky, and feverish. Nancy said he had a cold and was upset by the yellow pipes in the street where the mains are being fixed. He said he felt sad. There is still no consistent word recognition. Only a sporadic joyful awareness of some links. After a second Coke, and a flurry of making thank-you cards for the fish fry, Ray declared himself no longer sad and asked Nancy where they could go next.

9/14/95

Nancy reported much improvement in Ray at home since Dr. Walker changed his meds. He jokes about Dr. Walker. Second project, more facial gestalts in puzzle form. Frustrating. Two foot stamps, and two call outs. He worked with pastels and needed his red towel. More outbursts. During a final chat his questions seemed pressured, urgent.

9/27/95

Ray in an excellent frame of mind. Nancy said he'd been talking about coming for a half hour before. Much chat about home and meals and gardens and family, the things he likes to talk about to deal with his energy and to reassure himself. With "seasons" in pictures, Ray simply couldn't connect. He could name all the elements of a picture but couldn't make the abstract leap into the concept of season. He got a kick out of the exercise, just didn't make the connection. Still couldn't get the facial gestalts. Watched Nancy do it, and got the first one on second try, but couldn't do the rest. Finished the session with free drawings, back to somewhat perseverative lines and circles. Put a lot of energy into it.

10/25/95

Great spirits. Lots of chat to establish connections. Did better on facial gestalt puzzles. He would match well and then lose the matches and then improve. No consistency. A bottle was leaking on the desk. That caused Ray to wear thin, and he took a break. After, he did a satisfactory glue/collage of leaves on a fall tree. He only had one outburst with drippy glue, but pulled himself together with his red rag. Last project, free drawings. Trees were somewhat successful at first, then went back to loops. Ray proudly showed off his glued tree in his meeting.

11/8/95

Ray spoke of a visitor. With Nancy's help he described the similar work Jayne Miller did with him in her assessment for facilitated communication. Did glued word matches. The glue bottle caused two outbursts when Ray was frustrated.

Next we did body gestalt puzzles. He did rather well with these but was frustrated with slick paper. This was reinforced with drawn figures to which Ray and I added arms and heads, etc. He finished with a quick computer story. (Emphasis on computer for Jayne Miller.)

11/20/95

Ray in fine spirits, but disoriented by trip into building. (?) He is enjoying his word/picture matches but there doesn't seem to be consistent improvement in recognition. He did a turkey gestalt puzzle, mostly prompted. He painted over a turkey, and pumpkin, and kept relative connection with the shapes. Don't know if GD (3-4) is due to organic impairment, repressed process or "laziness" but it is a challenge to see if he can advance. Will go to a color book approach for readiness.

He turned on the monitor and inserted the disc for our dictated story. Won't use keyboard. (Jayne Miller recommends a scrapbook binder to facilitate conversation with Raymond.)

12/8/95

Raymond came in and hit the door. I diffused the hits by modeling them. Jayne Miller has suggested asking Ray for better ways to say Butt Out. He has found looking for alternative expressions amusing. Ray chatted about the holidays. His speech is notably more conversational and humorous. He asks his conversation starters but broadens the topics and becomes general. He is very good with brand recognition. Could do comparisons with words that look like brands. Ray colored in a self portrait, and then made 8 very successful collage xmas cards.

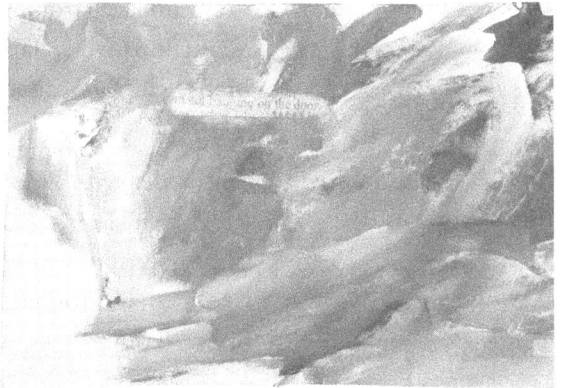

Raymond's painting "I'm not banging on the door."

1/3/96

We focused on word pages for the scrapbook. He recognized 20 out of about 60 word pictures (words underneath pictures). Ray wrote a poem for his book. It was

UP HERE

I took the TV and put it on the table.

I moved the furniture.

Raymond got sick in the stomach.

Raymond threw a fit.

It was bad.

Raymond then picked his nose. His nose bled.

He was screaming last night.

Raymond was yelling last night.

That was a bad move.

I told Raymond I had eaten all the lovely cookies that he had brought me for

Xmas. He laughed and said. "You pig." We all howled.

1/19/96

Ray came in in good spirits. Nancy said it cheered him up when he saw her come pick him up for art. He was apparently comfortable with the meeting with John O'Brien. (1/18/96)

He would wander in and remark on things said and engage various participants in tangential conversations. He enjoyed doing his word matches and pages. He colored in vehicles and enjoyed that. He did a free drawing in his circular movements. He called it snails. It looked like that and I added "antennae" and he liked that. (Aunt Mary airport poem.)

(Met with Nancy and Betty about activities of daily living issues.)

2/8/96

Worked extensive word pages. Wrote under words instead of reading print words. He enjoyed this but still doesn't demonstrate a grasp of the connection between the written word with picture and reading the words independently. Did gestalt recognition with large fruit pictures. He enjoyed painting them. Identified all but strawberry, maintained fruit shapes in painting except for grapes. Intense story Aunt Mary, Big Mao's, which he identified as a Chinese restaurant.

2/22/96

Good spirits. Enjoyed word pages. Recognized several vegetables to paint, even a cucumber. He enjoys Nancy's feedback. He did a free-form picture which he said after some questions was Nancy's garden. Did a story.

Did an impromptu "eye test" using his name in several sizes. He was able to identify each one.

3/13/96

Dr. Walker gave Ray Prozac. He is more even-dispositioned in the evening and can better predict an outburst, saying, "Don't do it, don't do it." But he was ataxic and off balance with his good disposition. He only had one outburst and it was minor, and he explained it shortly after and apologized. In his story he said he was happy. He talked about having a seizure in the bathroom.

He really enjoyed his story and he stayed on task with each activity longer than ever before. He was into things and rarely drifted. He incorporated some of his words into the dictated story. He even asked to draw again after the computer story. He was in no hurry to leave.

3/26/96

Ray was taken off Prozac. The instability and lability continued to increase. Dr. Walker had suggested Haldol increase. Betty said no. He had two rough weeks. He looked dark and unconnected. He was glad to be at art, but was not so comfortable. He has been asking at home when he can come back. His favorite part is stories.

He colored flower gestalts. He yelled when his pen lids wouldn't work. Did a name gestalt with his middle name backwards. He knew his forward name.

He wanted to talk his story a long time, but wasn't as free about speaking in sentences as he'd been the last visit.

4/15/96

Raymond has asked in times of stress when he could come back to art therapy so this must be providing some release for anxiety. Very tense at home; outbursts even at Raymond's meeting. Betty is upset and concerned about the moving out. R. says. "I don't want my stuff to go somewhere else."

I planned some gestalt paintings but before I got to the table Ray had the brush and water and proceeded to paint the table cover with relaxed free strokes. He was certain and comfortable and stopped his outbursts which had been more prominent than ever. "I'm relaxed," he announced, "and happy." He called the picture "fine, better" and promptly started a second one. It was more convoluted, less free. He called it "even better." He quickly did five more word match drawings, painting each one with dispatch. He was ready to break and then do the story. He was very excited about going to see the river. "I am going to get a kick out of this story, Gah!" He was really engaged, not stuperous like the Prozac made him. Nancy wondered if the Haldol he'd had before our session curbed the outbursts or if relaxing with the painting did.

4/29/96

Ray came in in splendid form. Nancy said, two really good days. He seemed calm and light, though Nancy saw some darkness in his face. He chatted and joked before working. He liked the pictures. It is like he knows the words are there, but is not too connected to them. He found the glue stick different. He almost yelled "f…" at it and stopped gracefully on the "f." He seemed pleased to have controlled that and went on.

He laughed out loud at the brand name page. "I am not going to be at all nervous, are you nervous?" he patted me jovially on the knee. We laughed about the Clorox for Colgate joke he'd played on a past story.

He enjoyed a balloon picture, remembering he'd seen balloons in the sky. He said a racehorse I presented looked like a dog. He painted it as a dog on the run with an unintended tongue extended. He called his last free painting a deer.

The images and ideas really flowed in his story. The rain blooming, the window joke. He worried about the oncoming storm but weathered it well.

5/13/96

Ray came in with Betty. He was only slightly out of kilter with the change in companion. He changed into long pants in the bathroom which required a fair amount of time and vocalization in the bathroom. Word pictures. He doesn't see black and white pictures at all well. Figure/ground issues. Painted several pictures that he liked including one he called TEFG. The letters he wrote didn't correspond to the ones on the paper. But it was a first step. Ray did the block poems and identified some words and stacked and moved the blocks. He seemed to enjoy the activity. He thought it interesting when I linked the words into phrases and would repeat each phrase. He said he'd like to do that again.

Gales of laughs with his poem. A strange dream sequence, humorous and rich. Monkey in a motel. Sheep go ribbit.

5/31/96

Fair mood. Only one partial outburst. Full of stories. He enjoys his word matches but isn't very successful. He is keen to stay inside a painted shape, but not discriminating about what is in the shape. He is eager to fill pages with color. He was not so keen on the blocks.

6/21/96

Used titles from previous poems for pictures which he painted. For some reason we got talking about the lens of the eye, and I drew a picture and explained it. He was very excited about this explanation and said, "I just love being here with you," as if hearing about things like this was a great relief. At times during the session he was a bit agitated and said about 4 times, "Would you just shut up." After he painted a while this agitation seemed to subside, and he declared himself to be "happy." The rest of our time, he acted happy. At the end he said to Nancy, "Would you just shut up," and I asked him quietly to apologize to her. He did, and seemed relieved. The story was a rollicking fun-fest. He got off on various parts and expressed interest in changes in his neighborhood and in varieties of fruits he enjoys.

7/3/96

Ray came in with Jim, then had to go out to Jim's car and get his drink. Nancy came to replace Jim. Ray raced through some numbered picture pages and seemed irritated by the process. He had five outbursts and seemed surprised by them. At one point he said he apologized to Jim. When I asked if he apologized for the outbursts at me he looked baffled and changed the subject. He painted number-oriented pictures. He seemed dull about them although he filled them. Ray was distracted during his story by a dry mouth.

7/18/96

Raymond came in a good mood. He wanted to talk. When I pulled out the old glued collage process he yelled out three times. He wasn't into gluing, and yelled about what bored him. He is dealing with deeper things in stories. He laughed at our attempts to understand a catch phrase he was trying to share with us that he and Jim use. He speaks about his day-to-day frustrations at home, and talks about ways to deal with disputes. He suggested that I sweep my office, and that he wanted to get papers for his mother to read.

"ABC is on 11. There were kids on ABC. They were looking at me...."

"The TV surprises me." Nancy and I later figured out that the catch phrase was, "Don't get mad, get glad."

8/1/96

Ray was practically effusive this day. He wanted to talk a blue streak. He made jokingly disparaging remarks about turkey that he'd had for lunch with Jim. He talked about home issues and laundry and time use. He asked about the condition of household appliances. He has an ever-expanding list of questions. We did facial expression identifications. He got "happy and sad" right off and differed from the word on the rest, although they were as likely descriptions of the ambiguous expressions shown. So he does recognize facial expressions. And these photos were in black and white, which has been a problem before.

He then did a large poster-size fish painting which he said he would use as his fish fry poster. We ended with a bang. He wanted to type. He did one letter at a time and enjoyed his nonsense sentence. He was not as engaged in the poem after that. The printer malfunctioned, and he was patient.

8/13/96

Ray did a glue-on menu for his fish fry. He enjoyed that. He did a full-body traced portrait to put up for the fish fry. He so enjoyed that that he had less energy for free paintings after that. He typed his title himself. Ox puno. "I went to St. Joe's. I won muffins. They cost $6.00 a piece."

9/17/96

(I moved my office between these two dates.)

Ray had a good day. I said something about knocking myself in the head and that really upset him. He reacted with an outburst. But we went on. He found our changed format word match initially frustrating. He tended to call s words – school, b words – baby, and c words – car. He didn't mind looking for the pictures but yelled out before finding elephant. He was aggravated by the markers, and needed his towel. His fine motor control wasn't at its best. This may have been due to the move.

He liked the "new computer." He clicked the mouse twice, a step ahead. He was aware of controlling his feelings and self reinforced and asked for reinforcement.

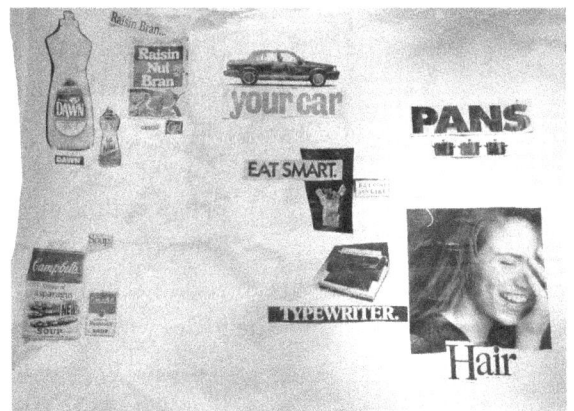

A word collage.

(9/30/96)

Meeting with Betty: "Raymond's been hollering out since the meeting. Jim S. comes at 8 a.m. Jim is feeling impatient. Mr. Atherton came home [rom hospital] Tues or Wed. That worked out well. He didn't have to have oxygen. He is getting better. He's on a 'bucketful' of meds. He has to hide to take them because that sets Ray off. He's at home, not going to work. I encourage him to keep moving.

'That's your cure for everything.' Ray's way was different. When my mother was ill he went to the hospital and watched all that happened. I couldn't let him stay alone. When Jim A. went to the hospital 2 1/2 years ago Ray asked Jim if he was going to die. Ray knew how ill he was this time.

"Ray and Owen came to the hospital. He sat there comfortably. He was happy for Jim to be home.

"He started acting out Saturday. 'He looks at me like he wants to kill me.' said Jim. Gerald said he felt that too. As Carolyn walked in Ray got started and we had to restrain him. He'd act out then get limp, then get started again then get limp.

"Day before he'd been carrying on. Jim said, 'Maybe when he hollers out give him a Haldol, and then another. Maybe we medicated him too soon. Owen said Raymond wanted to come home early.

"I knew then it was coming. He was holding in the rage and then he'd get started, and we'd pin him down over and over. It was getting pretty tiresome. He went to bed and there went the TVs. He never asked for help this time. The look on his face was somebody else.

" 'Let me up, I'll be good,' he'd say. Gerald would let him up because he can get him down. Gerald offered to stay the night. Gerald got up with him for some shouting out. He started then throwing the TVs and the lamp. We decided not to medicate him and let him fight it out. He'd scream and want to beat on Gerald. He just kept cussing.

"The Seven Counties thing has so confused me. All the mixed dates. Stacey doesn't have a clue.

"Nancy called Milt and Hope and you. Then he went to Owen's. When Owen came in the yelling stopped. Like turning a radio off. Raymond couldn't get his underwear on. Physically rattled. Every time he goes through a spell he loses a bit.

"He asks about Brian [Raymond's nephew] staying with us."

(Ray stayed with Owen for about a week during this crisis. Betty and I discerned three parts to the conflict. Transition anxieties – Brian and territory issues – and Jim A.'s illness.)

"My energy is shot. I've been edgy after the men all go to bed or to work.

Betty's optimism. "I do the doing, Nancy does the thinking."

"This time there was no sense that the crisis would ever be over. I am concerned about Jim Schrecker being able to handle Raymond. Raymond's been wanting me to help him with pajamas. 'I need help.'

"He used to go to his siblings' to spend the night. He doesn't want to stay the night with anyone now. Gerald offered to take him for a night out. He doesn't trust the meetings anymore. I want his personality to come back."

10/3/96

Ray has been staying with Owen since the crisis over the weekend. He is better. Gerald is talking about getting a duplex and setting Ray up there.

Ray enjoyed the wall words even though he was unusually ataxic in his movement. His gait was off and his look darker than lately. He made much less eye contact. I had made a birthday cake for him. He was glad for it and wanted to take it with him, wrapped for the trip home. When we painted he was unusually uncomfortable and shouted out seven times: when I introduced the sponge; twice when I helped him choose paints; and three times while painting, and when I asked if he wanted to name it.

He was so agitated while we did the story that I didn't suggest he type. He pushed questions with a lot of force as if the asking and repeating them offered him some contact and tranquility. During the story he continued to ask establishing questions and was more distracted than he has been since he started doing the stories.

10/24/96

Ray was identifying pictures of dogs as ducks. I don't know if he was teasing me or really saw them as such. He happily identified and read the word house. Green on black. I wondered if the color switch helped. The apple screen was green on a dark background.

He worked intensively on a card for Julie and Owen to celebrate their new baby. He paid attention to this task for 45 minutes. We also had a 30-minute conversation over Coke. It didn't bother him that he didn't do a story.

11/7/96

Did small pages of light letters on dark to see if that improves things. Babies. Dana's Katie and Owen's Grace. Ray was cheery and excited over the new babies. But a storm was brewing outside and he became tighter and began to suck on his lower lip. As we continued our activity, he started to yell. He was becoming more uncomfortable by the minute. I asked if he'd rather do a computer story than word pages. He said yes. It was hard for him to focus on the story. He yelled a few more times and then would try to self-reinforce. "You won't cancel me, Nancy?" "I am good. I am going to be better." "I want to talk about mother. She is being good. That makes me happy. Daddy is being good. Sometimes he is being bad. Beating on the door. Me, I am being good." Nancy shared that he'd not had a good day, and tension had built up since morning. After the story the rain let up a bit. I asked Ray if he wanted to draw, since that usually relieves tension. He worked at it but was yelling and having a hard time staying in control. His first piece was yellow pumpkins. He put a lot of energy into it and yelled several times. If I suggested anything, he yelled. Any deviation was a threat. His second piece was a large black piece about his Christmas TV. "Two more months." he reiterated. He reinforced about being relaxed several times, but then had to yell. The last picture was red Christmas trees. I opened the pens for him. Nancy called Jim, since Ray wanted to finish early. He threw down his wallet and yelled more. We went outside to wait. He yelled. Then he and Nancy got into her car to wait.

11/21/96

Ray came in full of chat. His gait was a bit ataxic but his humor was engaged. Lots of conversation, new babies, TVs, foods, etc. He looked at my face and made eye contact. He assured Nancy and me that he wouldn't fuss. No shout out ever. He mentioned early in the session that his dad was a lot better. He said this with warmth and enthusiasm and laughed out almost relieved. I wonder how much fear and grief has been connected to his dad's illness. A figure ground exercise was telling. He could see flowers and the "garden" (jungle) but couldn't see the parrot, or the monkey and lion who were easily identified by strong facial gestalts. A large crayon drawing, not taped down, with lots of pressure and moving about of the crayon did not elicit any yells. At one frustrated moment he informed me that he was not going to get upset. He wasn't upset that the computer was down, and went right on as I typed his story, about Miss Kitty (Raymond's cat). We went downstairs and he was delighted to see Jim arrive.

12/5/96

Ray was in finest fettle. He wished us happy holidays, he was light and had good color in his face. His gait was steadier and he was voluble and full of fun. With the word sheets, it is almost as if he pops into awareness and then out again. I can't tell if light on dark had improved anything.

Ray made five construction paper cards with the letters PBD repeated over them several times. Even with two breaks to do other things, he would come back to this activity. We made fold-up envelopes and he put a folded story in each one as a gift.

12/20/96

Ray was in a good humor. He enjoyed word references to Christmas and TVs. He enjoyed decorating a tree on the wall. He glued a number of various ornaments onto the tree. I had a paper chain for him to put on the tree, but he didn't want to do that, he wanted to see how I had made it. So we did that for a while. He did two watercolors. Only one minor negative during the painting. But he said several times, "I am not going to grump anymore."

Raymond continued to visit Julie for art therapy until winter of 1998.

Appendix F

Poems

We wanted to put quite a few of Raymond's poems in this book because they were a rich portrait of how Raymond viewed his personal world. The poems were dictated to Julie, the art therapist, in the form of conversations that Raymond generated, and Julie typed up rapidly. Raymond enjoyed counting out how many copies he wanted to take to relatives and friends after each poem was written.

You Make Me Nuts   December 29, 1997

You made so happy.
I got a Magnavox.
I got cable. Do you have it Nancy?
I'm not goin' to worry about any more?
I blew it out.
No I take it back, I got the end table.
For my TV
It came in a box, Julie, the TV.
It was big, 32 inch, the box.
I can't get the Styrofoam out of the box.
Can't hardly get it out.
Did you get one, Nancy?
Mitsubishi peanuts, Melt not in the hand.
Ohhh yeah.
It is on TV at night.
Snickerbars.
Gerald does, he ate a whole thing up.
Last night ago. I gave them to him.
Sorry you are so funny, Nancy.
I know what it is. Fresh candy.
In an aspirin bottle
It gave me a headache last night, your mother did.
Snickerbars. No.

I went to Ms. Kothen's and got peppermint candy, for Ms. Kothen
Don't want to forget my paintings Julie.
Mitsubishi peanutbutter cups.
Uh oh, I gotta tell Julie that, popcorn tins. From Nancy
$200 apiece.
I ate cheese popcorn.
Ate nuts. Caramel nut candy at Aldi's store.
They are going to move to Gardiner Lane.
Hurstbourne Lane, Aldi's
NO mother did.
Breckinridge lane.
Pecan pie.
Dr. Pepper, she got them at Kroger. Mother does.
Vicky went on a vacation. Ginny is in Milton's house.
When we pulled up. Ginny is going on a trip.
Did you go Nancy?
How was it, are you going back again?
How's your job doing?
How is the typing doing today, Julie?
Oatmeal
Daddy's a pig, oinkoink, Yeah.
Moo cow. He ate a whole thing up. Of oatmeal.
Milk, no milk jug. I drank a whole gallon of it.
You want some, Nancy?
I drink orange better, a whole glass of it.
How is your fruit doing?
You need a new calendar?
Ready for a cleanday. Reddy Electric, Daddy got it for me.
Eleven days. Dr. Daddy is going.
I am nice Nancy.
Talk. I like to talk to my friends. Best buddy.
Yeah.
Hot dog. Anchovies. Sausage with mushrooms. Pizza
Olives, green ones.
Fruit cocktail. Not on pizza.
Monkey.
Don't want to forget the paintings, dry enough.
Have to wait and see.

Monkey and the ape.
Zibbet. Willie loved camping
HE got a whiz bang out of it.
Too cold for me to go camping, Oh yeah.
Sleep in the bed tent, in it.

Sleep at night in the camper.
Deam lake. How is your swmming doing?
Daddy fishes.
Campfire. Smell it. Hot dogs. Roast the hot dogs.
Do you get one, Nancy?
Bout through.

Monkey

Monday January 6, 1997

Lions, shoes, snails,

Happy.

Ribbit.

Don't give me a heart attack, Julie!

Crickets say ribbet.

Going in the water.

I know I have a good imagination

Sibbet, Ribbet, Cwack Quack, Shibbet.

Ribbett.

The Church, It's breaking my heart.

Record Player, Neil the needle.

Play it. Uh Oh I broke it.

What time does your son do that?

CDs

Country Boy, Boogies.

Country Songs.

Cowboy Songs.

Country Music.

S Garden.

Vegetables, Green Beans.

I got a whole can of it. At home.

Pecan Pie. Carolyn makes that.

Raspberries. Don't give me a heart attack.

Fruit cocktail. I'm having a ball, too!

RC, Wow, I got two liters at the store.

I drink too much beer, I like it, Yes I does.

I love hot chocolate, a whole box full.

Don't give me a heart attack Nancy.

Funny!

Tea Kettle, Coffee Pot. ON the stove.

Coffee in the morning.

I am not wild, Nancy.

Daddy drinks coffee. Cream.

Nuts. Pecan Pie.

Mushrooms. Sausage.

Raspberries. Cheese.

Mushroom cheese.

Green Peppers. Anchovies.

Don't give me a hard way to go, Julie.

Banana Bread. Jim's a good cook.

Julie burns the stove too much. It's awful

Meatloaf, Meatloaf! It burnt, it went kaput again.

Gosh it's terrible. On the table.

 No, she's got a skillet.

That's weird, Yes!

Julie ate the meatloaf.

Owen has not eaten it, not yet!

Pear! Gaw, Get real.

Carolyn told me that, Get real.

On a plate. They are good and sweet.

Check book Wow, Goj do you love that?

Julie loved that.

I got a new TV table. A Magnavox.

Forty two inch TV. Well 32.

Ice skate. It like to watch it the best.

Oatmeal. Bran Flakes.

Snails, cattlefish. Soup.

Vegetable Soup

Pop Tarts. They're great.

Toast. Pop tarts toast.

Amanda eats them.

Aaron likes them.

Bedroom door. Jim's talking on the phone too much.

Baby. I know what it is, Grace.

Julie's Grace. Julie's a good feeder.

Grace lies down in Owen's bedroom too much.

She is in the bassinet. I know what it is.

Grace plays with her toys in the bedroom.

Baby bed toys.

I am smiling too much. I got a smile on my face.

My face got better.

Jim's car ran out of gas. It's his fault.

I Love You

Me, I love you.
I love my Mother.
And Dad.
I love my Dad.
I am sitting in the couch.
I am watching TV.
I am watching news.
It is on Channel 3
Movie.
Scary movie.
Monkey.
Cough drop.
Don't get me wrong, Nancy.
I be happy with it.
I broke the big screen TV.
It fell. It broke.
Knocked the end table over.
Knocked the phone over.
The TV where the couch is.
Snowman.
Making snow,
Rain.
Getting rain, too?
Go Away, the rain.
The sun came out.
Your's come out, too?
Come back another day.
Wash the windows.
Watch the sunset.
Moon.
In the sky.
My garage, car garage.
Driving in it.
Downhill.
I fall in the snow.

Yesterday morning.
Raspberries.
Strawberries.
Yogurt.
Strawberry yogurt, cookies.
Nike. Shoes.

No slamming the door today.
Marshmallows. Fruit cocktail.
Dessert. Pineapple juice.
Raspberry juice. Pineapple.
Dessert Pie. Pizza Pie.
Mr. Gatti's got it. Pineapple.
Peach yogurt.
Soft drinks. A whole box full.
Diet. Diet Rite.
Radio. Listening to music.
I love a blanket. The green.
Snowshoes.
Driving Owen's car. Station wagon.
Julie loves it.
Pop tarts. Amanda eats them all.
Jelly. Cookie scraps.
Start cookies. Fudge cookies.
Pineapple cookies.
Raspberry juice.
Vanilla cookies.
Apple juice.
Restaurant.
Micky D's.
Birdcage.
A new lamp.
Fish. Jim buys it too much.
Finger cookies. Amanda made them. She ate them.
Birthday cake. Pop tarts.
Raspberry juice.
Snail

Moving Furniture   February 6, 1997

Watch TV News.
David Letterman
I changed the channel.
Good Morning America.
Oprah Winfrey.
Statue. I don't know.
Wheel of Fortune.
Jeopardy. Alex Trebek.
Shave. My whiskers.
I did my own face.
I am not going to shout anymore.
Grapefruit juice.
Milk. Orange juice.
I like to drink it.
Don't be Picky, Nancy.
Book. Story Book.
I left the stories in Church, when I did the bulletins last week.
I took them to Dr. Strumpf.
Oatmeal Pizza Pie.
Sailboat.
Left the stories in Dr. Strumpf's box.
Peanut butter.
I eat it. I eat it on crackers.
Jelly. I eat it on peanut butter.
Sandwich. Peanut Butter and Jelly Sandwich
I take a bite. It makes me feel healthy.
SnacklePop. Cereal.
Banana.
Banana pudding. Yesterday.
Jim made it.
Pecan Pie
She is going to get a whiz bang out of it.
Schmarshmallow. Peach cobbler. Strawberries.
Raspberries. Cranberries. Fruit Cocktail.
Tuna fish.

My chair is not too close. I will move it up.
The desk.
Hotsy Totsy.
What's wrong with you Nancy?
I am not mad anymore.
Banana Bread. Jim makes it.
Don't cancel me, Nancy.
Brian got a new job. At Mr. Gatti's
He used to work at Little Caesar's
He's working late.
He likes his job.
Brian's going to get home at midnight.
He brings me pizza.
And Brian eats it.
I never get any.
The sun is asleep at night.
It is going to be dark at night.
Mother washes the dishes in the morning.
Drying dishes in the morning.
Mother does.
She cooks with them. The dishes.
Bakes cookies in the morning.
I did snack on those cookies.
Oatmeal. Oatmeal cookies.
Jelly cookies. Star cookies.
Monkey. In the water.
Sibbet.
A lion. Giraffe. Zebra in a cage.
Pet the animals.
Give Jim the carrots. To feed the animals.
Don't make me late, Nancy.?
Monkey. Vegetable.
Jimmy eats vegetables.
Pat, Pet.
Nancy, don't scare me.
I am not tense anymore.
It's enough.

I Moved Furniture, I Did!   February 19, 1997

I watched TV.

Ice cream. Marshmallow, Ice cream.

Cupcakes, with Chocolate icing.

Oatmeal. Chocolate chips.

Pizza Pie.

Fruit Cocktail.

Raspberries.

Foot TV. 200-Foot TV

Pizza Pie.

Jim is going to Brenda's tonight.

He is not going to make it tonight.

He is going out to eat tonight.

Banana Bread. Jim made it for Brenda.

Raspberry. Watch out!!

Dessert Pie. Jelly Pie.

Peach Pie. Apple Pie.

Anchovies. It's allowed, Nancy.

Tomatoes.

Raspberry.

Peach Cobbler.

Banana Bread.

She weighs one pound, Grace.

Oat Bran, she eats.

Baby food. Sweet baby food.

For Owen's Julie's baby.

Applesauce. Julie Feeds her.

Ice Cream. The baby is going to get sick.

If I give her a whole gallon full.

A bucket full.

Jump on it. Jump on the ice cream.

And get drunk.

The baby would throw it up.

She would throw a fit.

I'd throw a pillow in the window.

At the baby bed.

No, she's going to tear her toys up.

Sometimes. No, she swells up in her hands.

She eats her arm up. She biting with teeth.

Baby teeth. Owen broke her teeth.

Julie Broke her tooth.

She went to the dentist.

The baby is getting baby teeth.

I got the phone broke for Julie

I got to tell Julie that the battery is dead.

Julie's phone ate the battery up.

Marshmallow. Cucumber.

Green pepper.

No anchovies.

Pizza pie with anchovies.

Tomatoes.

Mr. Gatti's. Jim goes.

I gave Brian a message off the phone machine.

His work wanted him to come in early.

Mushroom

Brian makes a pizza with mushroom.

Sometime he likes that.

Anchovies.

Jennie got an awful cold. She lost her voice last night.

I gotta show Jennie that.

Is she coming this evening?

You want me to give her this story tonight?

How's your phone book doing?

What time do you use it?

I went to Kroger today with Julie.

I got bologna.

Julie loves it.

I fed Susie a whole pound full.

Chocolate milk. Orange juice.

I've got one at home.

What am I going to do when I get home tonight?

Go ahead write it. I got enough!

Peanut Butter Jar, Jam Jar, Snicklefritz

June 3, 1997

Sourcream

Olive pizza. Anchovies. Tomatoes. Onions.

Stick it in the mouth.

Tasty excellent pizza.

Mushroom.

Soft drink dispenser.

I'll drink a whole gallon of Pepsi.

Can smasher. I did.

I moved furniture. The TV's moved.

Oatmeal cookies.

How's your desk doing Nancy.

No problem. Paper work. Gaah chew.

I'm not going to be fussy anymore.

I be patient.

I be happy.

Chocolate chip cookies.

Marshmallows. Stick em in the mouth.

Jam bucket. Tools in it.

Neisy got a new garden. Tonight. Bingo!

I am going to see it tonight.

Neisy got tomatoes, Bingo!

Raspberry soup.

Owen didn't cook last night.

He's not home. He's on vacation.

Daddy is going to the doctor.

Pumpkin pie. Meemaw done that.

Whipped cream on pie.

You're darn right. Memaw's a good cook.

Meemaw made meatloaf last night. Excellent!

I know what it is, dog biscuits.

Give me a break.

The coffee shop has dog biscuits, Gaah.

Poplar Level Road,

Heitzman's coffee shop.

$200 a piece. I can't afford that.
For Susie. One pound of dog biscuits.
She liked it. She ate the whole thing up.

Julie Had Coffee

Julie had Coffee
Owen's a coffee drinker, too.
I know what it is.
Owen changed his room yesterday.
Oh, I'm gonna miss him.
Susie was going to the bathroom yesterday.
Daddy's smoking a pipe in the bedroom.
Daddy's going to get a kick out of it.
Bubble bath. Oh shoot.
Smoking pipe, like bubbles out of a bubble pipe.
I took the pressure off of Daddy.
Whoo Whooo Whoooo!
It makes me happy to do that.
It made Daddy sad. He was crying yesterday. Poor baby.
Chill out Julie.
He was a cry baby.
The mother gets sad sometimes.
Smiling on my face.
Wind on my face. I got a smile on my face.
I am going to be surprised in my room.
Small TV It's going to be a Magnavox TV. It's coming in the mail, in a box.
You want some Julie?
I am going to be happy with it.
I am not going to tear up stuff anymore.
I am in a good mood today.
Daddy let me use his telephone.
I called a wrong number
Stopped the bill. Phone bill
Won't charge for a wrong number.
Momma got a new humidifier.
It brings air in the basement.
Walmart got it.
Circuit City they had it too.
H.H. Gregg got it.
I'll be happy with it. I am going to be happy with it.

Fan motor in the basement.

My air conditioner is in the closet in the bedroom.

Fan belt. Gaaah Choom.

I know what it is. The mirror in Jim's car.

My Gerald fixed it for me.

Do you need a mirror fixed, Nancy?

Fan blade on the car. Fluid, fluid in the car. Brake fluid.

Brian's got a new girlfriend.

She's got a new apartment.

Brian got an apartment. I don't know.

I did not ask.

Scheuuu.

I know what it is. Watching TV in a motel

Channel TV Cable channel.

A Disney movie. On the Disney Channel.

Murder She Wrote, on the Disney channel.

On channel 32 Oprah Winfrey.

News at 4:00 o'clock

End table Cheew.

I've got a big lamp on the headboard of the bed.

TV on the Button Box in the Bedroom, next to the computer TV

It's going to be a new one. TV table,

Gaah Cheeeew.

Small lamp on the dresser.

I get out of bed in the morning.

Do you do that Nancy? Cheeeew.

I get dressed.

I've got a green blanket. Meemaw gave it to me.

My green blanket is orange.

I keep warm. Snuggle on the bed.

Quilt blanket. It is red and green.

You need one, Nancy?

Miss Kitty, She got sick last night.

We threw her out.

My mother got angry last night.

She was grouchy.

She was upset last night.

Don't worry about it. She's not upset today.

She's in a good mood today.

A happy mood.

I am going to borrow your car today, Nancy.

I 've got a computer in the TV room.

My kids messed it up.

Carolyn Stansbury messed it up.

I'm going to see Carolyn tomorrow.

Waffle toast, with butter on it.

Eating it on a plate with a fork.

Spooning it in the mouth.

I am ready for dishing the pie. Eating her curds and whey.

The dish ran away with the spoon.

I gonna be ready to find out.

Chocolate cake. He was ready to cut the cake.

And the dish ran away with the spoon.

Butter fly

Pumpkin pie.

Over the moon, Up the sky.

Gave the dog a bone to make it laugh.

Monkey pie

Pop goes the weasel.

Jumped over the moon.

Moonshine

March 24, 1997

Night time. The moon.

Easter Bunnies.

Give me a break.

Easter eggs.

Easter Baskets.

Chocolate Bunnies.

I ate a whole basket of it.

A whole basket of jelly beans.

Don't give me a lot of trouble.

The little black ones, oh wow.

Honey jelly beans, wow gosh.

I know what it is, a green basket.

Daddy's going to enjoy it.

You know what the kind is, chocolate rabbit.

You know what it is.

Don't get me wrong, Nancy.

It is going to have my name on it.

Blue Easter eggs, Blimey, Oh God.

Pineapple. I'm trying to think.

I'm telling you Nancy.

Marshmallow, a whole basketful.

Green Jelly beans.

You know what kind it is,

Purple jelly beans.

Mom's going to get a kick out of it.

She' going to get them at the store.

Chocolate eggs. Oatmeal eggs. Gaaah, give me a break.

No Easter cookies.

Chocolate bunnies. Chocolate eggs.

I'm happy. I am in a good mood.

Eat it. In the mouth. Get real.

I do want to eat it with my teeth, gaaah.

Give me a break.

Marshmallow. Easter bunny bag.

Chocolate rabbit.

Red jelly beans whoooo.

I know what it is, pumpkin pie. I'll be my guest.

Have you been to Evansville, Nancy?

Whipped cream, I could eat it all day.

I Had a Great Time   August 24, 1997

I've been working hard.

Sweeping, back yard.

You do that, too?

How's your raking doing?

What time did you rake it?

Oatmeal

Don't be nit picky.

Mushroom.

Don't do that, Nancy.

Nope, chill out.

No. Owen told me that.

Mushroom pie.

Did you buy one?

The chair is going to fall today.

I went out with Cliff today.

We went to the bowling alley.

Bowling alley was busy.

Jennie is coming tonight.

She is going to play pinochle with me.

Fruit cocktail.

Ice tea jar. A bucket full of tea. A whole gallon of it.

In the orange cooler.

How's the dishwasher doing.

How's the house doing.

Pour down rain. I was at Denise's

Don't go too fast.

Pizza pie.

Need some more again.

Dad's car squeaks. It's got dirt in it.

It's got mush brakes. It makes a funny noise.

Gerald is going to do it.

Chocolate chip cookie. M&Ms jar.

Not in the hand

Melt in the mouth, Shew!

Sweet teeth. Wooden teeth.

Nobody has them.

George Washington Butch

George Bush in Washington. President Bush.

Shopping the phone Bill

Reagan.

President Bush on the Show.

President Bush got a trophy on TV.

He won something on TV

I know what it is. George Washington Bush.

President Clinton's show. Saw it the other day.

A soap bubble.

Changed the channel with the remote control.

I am going to be jumping up and down, Nancy.

I know what it is. Dan Rather's show, the National News.

Wheel of Fortune.

Pig. Rerun.

Channel 32 News. Liz Everman.

Saw the Belle on the news, win the trophy.

She sunk. Swim. It's too cold for me.

It makes me throat. Float. I am going to get sick in the pool.

I am going to be surprised, Nancy.

President Bush was playing ball on the show. Yeah.

Football. He's playing for Hikes Point. Two games.

I saw him on Forty One. He was the coach.

He had gold teeth.

Wooden teeth. President Bush.

Football coach. President Reagan's flag. Stick flag.

He was singing with the football coach.

Up in the air. The flag. The TV sang.

Happy birthday to you, Happy birthday to you. Happy birthday dear Mom, Happy
    birthday to you. . . .

Strawberry on the ground.

Cut grass. How's your grass doing.

Time you cut it, Nancy?

Mom cuts the grass.

Oatmeal pie.

I am not going to argue again . . .

Basement.
Washerdryer. Nancy, did it. Washing?
How's your washer doing?...
Monkey going in the bath room.
Going in the bath tub. Takes a shower.
Toilet paper. Cat playing with it. Good cats.
I know what it is.
Wasting the toilet paper in your bathroom.
Called the plumber. Started the toilet up.
Making a mess in the bath room
Your cat. . . .

Monkey

September 8, 1997

Bean soup. I don't like bean soup.

Raspberry soup.

Macaroni. Jim fixes it. In the oven.

Cheese. Macaroni cheese. Two cups of cheese.

A whole pan full. Munch on it. Hot.

I like it hot. Eat it.Crackers. Crackers and cheese.

I know what it is.

A grilled cheese sandwich. Butter on it.

I like it on a plate.

Milk and cheese sandwich. Green peppers.

Whole bunch of it.

A pan full in the garden.

I ate tomatoes. Shoney's.

Taylorsville Rd. Hikes Point.

At the bowling Alley.

I won two games.

Jennie was not there. Today.

She's gone out of town. I did not ask.

What is wrong with me, Nancy?

Jennie's Mark went with her.

They went to Bunco. It is on Sunday.

I don't know whose house.

Played ball. Jennie. She likes to play soccer ball.

Camera. Roll of film. Not yet taken to be developed. Twelve pictures.

Drug Emporium. I got shampoo.

I know what it is, bug spray.

$8 apiece.

Bugs in the bedroom.

Spraying in the bedroom.

A whole gallon of it. They'll eat my house up.

Ms. Kitty got the bugs. Fleas.

Ms. Kitty got sick because of the bug spray.

She got sick in Daddy's couch.

It made him mad.

The mother cleaned it all up.

Don't want to forget to tell her that they were eating the room up, the bugs.

Roof's leaking. From the gutter.

Down the drain. When it's starting to rain.

Up 'ere.

A leaf blew over.

I am going to be lucky, Nancy.

Answer the door. Surprise come. Real screen TV.

For my room.

14' that operates it. I am not going to break it anymore.

No. Daddy told me that. Coming to my door.

Ring the door bell. Jumping up and down. Be happy.

Chill out, Nancy.

I am not fussing anymore. I am so good, so good.

I am not grumpy anymore. I am better.

Know what it is. It is going to be my birthday, October 4th.

Three more months till Christmas.

Chocolate cake, for my birthday.

The mother bakes it. It is going to be ice cream. You wanna come? . . .

Apple pie, all weekend. Twelve pies, I stick it in the oven. Carolyn made it. Cathy
    brought the apples.

Mom brought a whole basket full from an apple tree in Cathy's yard. . . .

Sustaining members of Raymond's group who participated in production of this book.

Cindy Bayes

Cindy likes to say she entered the field at 20 months old when a beautiful baby sister who was later profoundly labeled came home. Having been blessed with a loving supportive family and good natural supports, Cindy learned to view the world through possibilities, rather than disabilities. She has worked as a case manager with the state of Florida Developmental Disabilities; placing foster children with special needs for the state of Kentucky; and as a program director at Seven Counties Services for the past 20 years. Cindy administers various community-based supports.

Julie Cole

An interest in too many things led Julie Cole to become an expressive therapist. She has continued an interest in many things. Those things made her learn about issues that affect the lives of people with marginalizing situations, such as disabling conditions. That prompted Julie to get involved both professionally and personally with a lot of people with disabilities. This led to her involvement in Raymond's group and to advocating for other friends. In addition to ghosting this book for Betty and the group, she has also written a novel, *Getting Life,* about a woman with disabilities working toward a more independent life.

Hope Leet Dittmeier

Hope started her career as a teenager working in a private institution for people with developmental disabilities. It was there that she began to ask the question, "What would it take for people to live ordinary lives in lieu of this?" Hope has spent the last 30 years trying to find the answer to that question. It was in a professional capacity, as a consultant committed to helping networks and service systems better support people identified as challenging, that Hope met Raymond and his family. It was as a neighbor, friend and advocate that she stayed around for years. It was Raymond and his family that taught her more about the answers to "what it would take" than anyone else she has ever met. Hope continues to use current work as the founder and director of Realizations, a grassroots agency with a mission to: Partner with people with disabilities to plan, create, and sustain custom supports that promote typical, socially valued lifestyles.

Hope is married to her high school sweetheart and has two incredible children. She is a student of Unity Truth Principles.

Linda McAuliffe

Linda McAuliffe is a Training Manager in Kentucky's Division of Mental Retardation. She came into Raymond's life as a case manager in 1992, recruited by Tim Estes to be in that role. At that point, she had approximately eight years of experience in the field of intellectual/developmental disabilities both in institutional settings and community-based supports. She found the experience of being a part of Raymond's circle so different from traditional case management, and so much more effective – best described as person-centeredness in action. As her professional roles changed, she remained a part of the circle. When she was self-employed she had a paid role in Raymond's life as well, which included accompanying him to art therapy with Julie. When she moved on to a job with the state, she continued to be part of the circle and offered insight and assistance when possible in navigating the service system. She considers her time with Raymond, his family, and his circle as one of the most educational and life-affirming experiences of her 23-year career.

Milton Tyree

Milt has enjoyed numerous opportunities through the years to develop personal relationships with people who have disabilities and their family members. He has more than 25 years of experience in the design, development, and provision of supports and services intended to promote participation of people with disabilities within valued aspects of everyday life. He has worked in a number of capacities including teaching, curriculum development, consulting, and program administration. His real passion is in the area of personal advocacy. Milt currently works for the Human Development Institute at the University of Kentucky.

Carolyn B. Wheeler

A native Kentuckian, Carolyn B. Wheeler has devoted her professional life to efforts which support people with disabilities to have full and meaningful lives in the community. While she has a Master's degree in Special Education, her work has focused on helping people plan for the future, with a specific emphasis on transition planning from high school to adult life. Through her work at the Human Development Instrument at the University of Kentucky, Carolyn was instrumental in the development of the Kentucky Hart-Supported Living Program, the promotion of Person-Centered Planning practices and supported self-employment for people with significant disabilities. Carolyn has developed an area of expertise in estate planning and is now a Special Care Planner with the MassMutual Financial Group. Through this venue, she assists families in creating a safe and secure future for their families.

www.ingramcontent.com/pod-product-compliance
Lightning Source LLC
Chambersburg PA
CBHW081148270326
41930CB00014B/3076